Brain Tumor Guide for the Newly Diagnosed

Tenth edition

Dr. Henry Friedman and Dr. Linda Liau reviewed and approved the contents of this guide.

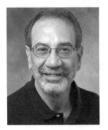

Henry S. Friedman, MD, is deputy director of the Preston Robert Tisch Brain Tumor Center at the Duke University Medical Center in Durham, North Carolina. An internationally recognized neuro-oncologist, Dr. Friedman has a long-standing career in the treatment of children and adults with brain and spinal cord tumors. He has written hundreds of research articles, and his work has been showcased on several segments of the CBS program *60 Minutes*. Dr. Friedman strongly believes that there is hope for patients who are being treated for brain cancer.

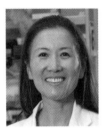

Linda Liau, MD, PhD, is the director of the UCLA Comprehensive Brain Tumor Program at the Ronald Reagan UCLA Medical Center in Los Angeles, California. She is a neurosurgeon with a clinical expertise in intra-operative functional brain mapping and imaging for resection of brain tumors. Dr. Liau's research is focused on the molecular biology of brain tumors, gene therapy, immunotherapy, and brain cancer vaccines. Her work has been published in journals and textbooks and has been highlighted on several television shows.

Copyright © 2016 by the Musella Foundation
for Brain Tumor Research & Information, Inc.

The Musella Foundation
1100 Peninsula Boulevard, Hewlett, NY 11557
888-295-4740   www.virtualtrials.com

ISBN 978-0-9899740-0-4

Brain Tumor Guide for the Newly Diagnosed

An up-to-date and essential guide to

Tools for getting organized

Understanding brain tumors

Your medical team

Surgery, radiation, chemotherapy, and tumor treating fields

Insurance management

Al Musella, DPM

Tenth edition

The Musella Foundation
for Brain Tumor Research & Information, Inc.

This book is sponsored in part by generous grants
from Genentech, Novocure, and the
Richard M. Schulze Family Foundation.

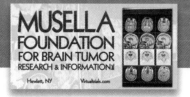

Table of contents

Introduction

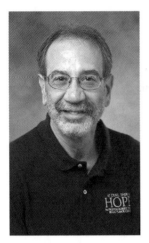

Henry S. Friedman, MD

If you have this book in your hands, it is possible that you or someone close to you have just received one of the biggest shocks of your life: the diagnosis of a brain tumor.

And as if that shock were not enough, let me add another: You now have to make immediate and important decisions about your brain tumor treatment.

The medical team who made the diagnosis will provide advice and guidance.

But because so many options exist — what doctors to choose, where to be treated, what treatments are available, what clinical trials can be entered — you need to become as informed as possible as soon as possible in order to make the best and most rational decisions.

The goal of ***Brain Tumor Guide for the Newly Diagnosed*** is to provide you, your family, and your friends with a basic primer of the "brain tumor" terrain. As the subtitle promises, this book provides tools for getting organized and information about your medical team and treatment. This book can be a vital first resource as you begin the fight against your brain tumor, by providing context for the world of brain tumor treatment.

A special feature of this book is that it is written with explicit reference to the virtualtrials.com website run and managed by the Musella Foundation for Brain Tumor Research and Information. The virtualtrials.com website was begun in the 1990s in order to list clinical trials and host online support groups for brain tumor patients. Since then, the website has grown steadily. There were over 500,000 visitors in the past year, from 224 different countries. For many people, the website has become an essential portal to brain tumor information and a place of shared experience. The website lists brain tumor centers, hosts and manages online support groups, keeps an up-to-date catalog of brain tumor clinical trials, and describes current and experimental brain tumor therapies. The website also provides links to, and actually gives, financial assistance.

This tenth edition of *Brain Tumor Guide for the Newly Diagnosed* is full of up-to-date links to different parts of the virtualtrials.com website and to other important websites. For some of these links, a QR code is provided for immediate access to a website by any smart phone with a camera and a QR reader app. QR reader apps are available for free from smart phone app sources.

A final word. Although it might feel otherwise right now, you are not alone. However difficult your next months or years will be as you fight your brain tumor, there are others who have lived through the experience and have a lot to share with you. Please reach out. There is a community that can support you — that *wants* to support you — beginning with the wonderfully resourceful Musella Foundation.

We wish you peace and health. ●

Henry S. Friedman, MD
Preston Robert Tisch Brain Tumor Center
Duke University Medical Center
Durham, North Carolina

Brain Tumor Guide for the Newly Diagnosed

Some notes about this edition

Internet links

This tenth edition of the ***Brain Tumor Guide for the Newly Diagnosed*** contains many up-to-date Internet links — to different sections of the virtualtrials.com website of the Musella Foundation and to other websites.

Due care has been taken to ensure that the Internet links are accurate. But as we know, such links are sometimes changed by the organizations that originally posted them.

At the virtualtrials.com website of the Musella Foundation, there is a separate webpage on which all the website links in this book are routinely kept up to date. To access that page to see a complete listing of the website links in this book, go to: www.virtualtrials.com/booklinks.cfm.

Glossary words

The page-bottom glossary definitions of some words come from the National Cancer Institute's online ***Dictionary of Cancer Terms,*** a resource with 7500 entries related to cancer and medicine.

The National Cancer Institute is part of the National Institutes of Health, which is one of 11 agencies that compose the Department of Health and Human Services in the United States.

Access to the ***Dictionary of Cancer Terms*** is available at the National Cancer Institute website (www.cancer.gov/dictionary).

Survivor stories

The survivor stories in this book are real but have been edited for this book format in order to highlight general themes and the specific interests of book chapters in which they appear. You can find the full stories for these survivors — as well as stories for other survivors — at the virtualtrials.com website of the Musella Foundation (www.virtualtrials.com/survive.cfm).

The Musella Foundation is deeply appreciative of all the people who have shared their stories at our website and in this book. Please share your story, too.

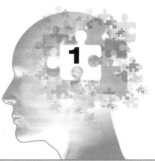

Chapter 1
Where, when, how, and why me?

Whether or not it was a loss of physical balance that led you to be diagnosed with a brain tumor, surely a loss of emotional balance quickly followed.

Every day, over 100 adults will be diagnosed with a primary brain tumor and many more will be diagnosed with a cancer that has spread to the brain from someplace else in the body, such as the lung or breast. Each year, thousands of parents will hear those two devastating words — brain tumor — in regards to their children.

There is no known cause of most brain tumors starting in the brain. There are indications that genetic factors or exposure to toxic chemicals or ionizing radiation may contribute to the formation of brain tumors. However, it is important to remember that you and your loved one did not do anything to cause the brain tumor and that each person and each brain is different.

There are over 100 kinds of primary brain tumors, some very rare. However, not all brain tumors, or even all malignant brain tumors, are invariably fatal. With surgery, radiation therapy, and **chemotherapy,** some types of tumors respond very well to therapy and may even be cured. While many of the more common tumors, such as **gliomas,** are not typically cured by surgical resection, there are more long-term survivors now than ever before, as new treatments have been introduced.

You will have a lot of important decisions to make with this medical conditon. You can make them yourself, or you can select a loved one or a team of loved ones to advocate for your care and treatment and to help you make important decisions. Not only will you have to make choices between treatment options presented to you, but you and your

---

Chemotherapy (KEE-moh-THAYR-uh-pee): *Treatment with drugs that kill cancer cells.*
Glioma (glee-OH-muh): *A cancer of the brain that begins in glial cells (cells that surround and support nerve cells).*

advocate may have to actively seek out options that your immediate medical team might not have access to.

To read survivor stories of people with brain tumors at the virtualtrials.com website of the Musella Foundation, go to: www.virtualtrials.com/survive.cfm.

Starting now

We are here to help you sort through various treatment options and to be a resource for you so that you can further understand your disease.

You must learn to question what you are told initially and, as treatment plans are put into place, to ask what qualifying factors your diagnosis and treatment plan are based upon.

You must also seek out the foremost expert advice.

Typically, your physician will have a treatment plan to discuss with you following your initial diagnosis. This plan may include a referral to a **neuro-oncologist** or neurosurgeon for a consultation regarding treatment options — such as surgery, radiation, chemotherapy, or enrollment in a clinical trial (more on clinical trial enrollment later).

While in some cases circumstances are such that emergency surgery is the only immediate option due to brain swelling or risk of acute brain injury, typically there is ample time to seek a second opinion and gather more information that can assist in your decision-making process.

The initial diagnosis is often stated as a brain lesion. A lesion is an abnormal tissue from disease or trauma; basically, there is something different about your brain, and a part of it does not look like normal tissue. Further testing, by means of brain imaging, is usually ordered to get a better idea of the size, location, and impact of the tumor, as well as locating any cancers in other parts of the body. It takes experience to be able to see some of the subtle differences in scans done by **magnetic resonance imaging (MRI)**

Neuro-oncologist (NOOR-oh-on-KAH-loh-jist): *A doctor who specializes in diagnosing and treating brain tumors and other tumors of the nervous system.*

Magnetic resonance imaging (mag-NEH-tik REH-zuh-nunts IH-muh-jing): *A procedure in which radiowaves and a powerful magnet linked to a computer are used to create detailed pictures of areas inside the body. These pictures can show the difference between normal and diseased tissue.*

1

or by **computed tomography (CT)**. A second opinion from an experienced doctor or medical team that frequently deals with brain tumors may change the initial diagnosis, in terms of either tumor type or grade, and thus may change your treatments. An MRI alone can be inconclusive (it may not be a tumor at all), making a thorough examination of all of your symptoms, and when possible, a **biopsy**, vital to your diagnosis.

The most important factor in your care will be the experience of the medical team treating you. If possible, ask for a second opinion from an expert source, preferably a major brain tumor center that is familiar with advanced forms of diagnosis and treatment of brain tumors. Also, ask for a **neuropathologist** experienced in brain tumors to review your biopsy. In many cases, brain tumor centers can coordinate your treatment (radiation and chemotherapy) with doctors more local to you, so that extended stays near the brain tumor center may not be necessary.

Your primary physician or oncology (cancer) specialist may not be familiar with the advances being made in the treatment of brain tumors. If your medical care team cannot answer your most pressing questions or is unwilling to consult on your behalf with available brain tumor experts, you must seek out further information and reliable sources for care, such as those found within major brain tumor centers. Many of these specialized centers will allow you to submit your MRI and CT scans, as well as biopsy specimens, for further examination directly without a referring physician.

The brain tumor neurosurgeons and team members at these brain tumor centers perform over 50 brain surgeries annually (some as many as five per week) and may offer the most technologically advanced procedures with higher rates of survival. Your choice of surgeon and treatment team can profoundly affect the outcome of your care.

If knowing your enemy (type and grade of tumor) is indeed half the battle, then having the tools to employ a strategy — a strategy for life — is equally important. Brain tumors can change, grow, and recur, so it is important to be organized and knowledgeable about your tumor's makeup and location, your medications and their side effects, and symptoms

---

Computed tomography scan (kum-PYOO-ted toh-MAH-gruh-fee skan): *A series of detailed pictures of areas inside the body taken from different angles. The pictures are created by a computer linked to an x-ray machine.*

Biopsy (BI-op-see): *The removal of cells or tissues for examination by a pathologist. The pathologist may study the tissue under a microscope or perform other tests on the cells or tissue.*

Neuropathologist (NOOR-oh-puh-THAH-loh-jist): *A pathologist who specializes in diseases of the nervous system. A pathologist identifies disease by studying cells and tissues under a microscope.*

you might expect throughout your treatment. It is equally important to maintain an on-going, open dialogue with your medical care team. Physicians rarely engage one another in the type of dialogue patients often assume is transpiring on their behalf. Being organized can assist you by ensuring all of your team members are up-to-date with current information at the time of your appointments and consultations. You and your advocate team must become your own primary care manager!

How to use this guide

This guide is made available to help you understand some of the common decisions you will be facing. It will answer some of the questions frequently asked by patients and care-givers and connect you with a support community. Additionally, it will help you get organized so that you can best advocate for the quality of care you need and deserve. Most importantly, this guide provides you with information on tumor types, the most current treatment options, and how to find major brain tumor treatment centers.

On the following two pages, there is a flowchart of the key messages in this book, linked to the chapters in which these messages are elaborated. This flowchart is intended to help reinforce what you need to start thinking about right now. If you pay attention to only one thing in this guide, pay attention to this flowchart.

Wherever possible, resource links to further online information have been provided for your convenience. Just type a URL web address into an Internet browser, or scan the QR codes in this book with a smart phone, or click a URL web address if you are reading an electronic version of this book. ●

If you ever have any questions or comments, please feel free to call us at the Musella Foundation at 888-295-4740 at any time between 10:00 AM and 6:00 PM ET Monday through Friday, and between 10:00 AM and 1:00 PM ET Saturday and Sunday. You can also submit questions by means of our website. Go to: www.virtualtrials.com.

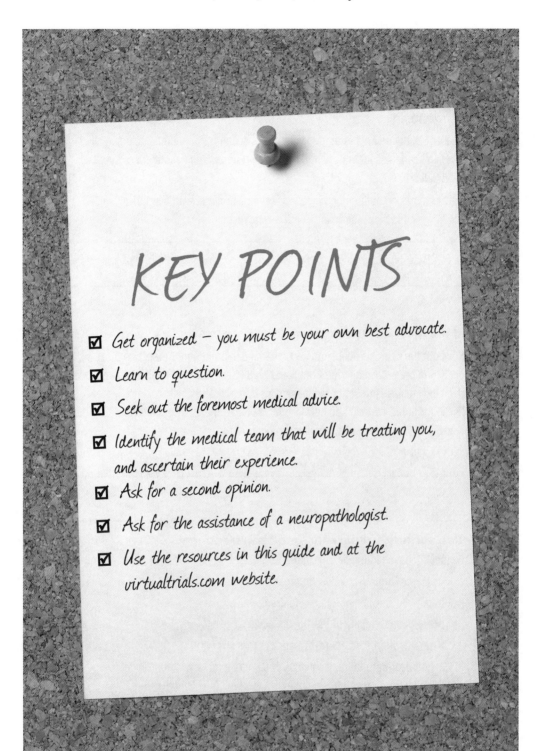

KEY POINTS

☑ Get organized – you must be your own best advocate.

☑ Learn to question.

☑ Seek out the foremost medical advice.

☑ Identify the medical team that will be treating you, and ascertain their experience.

☑ Ask for a second opinion.

☑ Ask for the assistance of a neuropathologist.

☑ Use the resources in this guide and at the virtualtrials.com website.

Starting now:
A guide to the *Brain Tumor Guide for the Newly Diagnosed*

Chapter 2

Get organized.

Request all documents related to your diagnoses and treatments, including all imaging scans and laboratory and pathology reports, and keep them organized in a binder.

Consider making audio recordings of your appointments with a smart phone and/or going to all appointments with a companion.

Chapters 3 and 4

Find the most advanced specialized care available to you.

Seek out the neurosurgeons most experienced in brain tumor resection at a dedicated brain-tumor center. Dedicated brain-tumor centers have advanced pathology facilities to better diagnose your tumor, better ability to store tumor tissue for future testing, and better familiarity with the latest science and advanced diagnostic and surgical techniques.

Chapter 5

Before surgery, prepare for long-term treatment.

Request genetic testing of your tumor tissue.

Ask how your tumor tissue will be preserved.

Ask about implantation of Gliadel wafers during surgery.

Ask about the availability of the Optune device.

If you are not offered standard-of-care therapy, ask why.

Standard-of-care therapy consists of surgery with or without Gliadel implantation, followed by radiation therapy plus the chemotherapy drug Temodar, followed by maintenance chemotherapy with Temodar plus alternating electric field therapy (the Optune device).

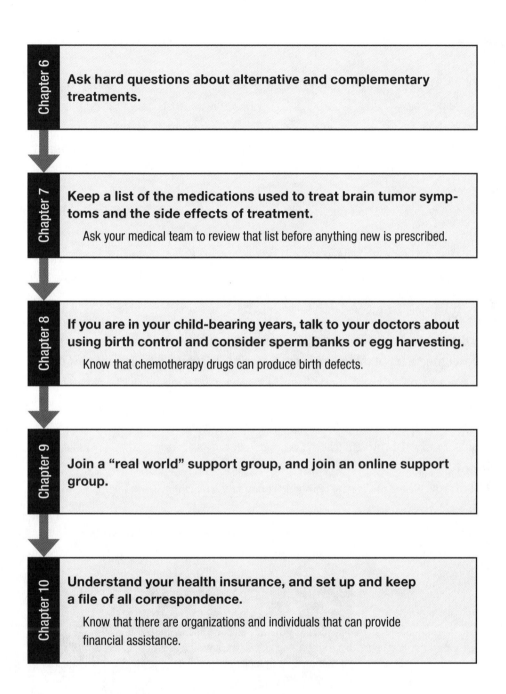

Chapter 6

Ask hard questions about alternative and complementary treatments.

Chapter 7

Keep a list of the medications used to treat brain tumor symptoms and the side effects of treatment.

Ask your medical team to review that list before anything new is prescribed.

Chapter 8

If you are in your child-bearing years, talk to your doctors about using birth control and consider sperm banks or egg harvesting.

Know that chemotherapy drugs can produce birth defects.

Chapter 9

Join a "real world" support group, and join an online support group.

Chapter 10

Understand your health insurance, and set up and keep a file of all correspondence.

Know that there are organizations and individuals that can provide financial assistance.

Survivor story #1

It started with small things in 1999, mostly visual. My wife thought I was experiencing a stroke.

I called my doctor at home on a Sunday. He had a scan set for Wednesday, my wife and I saw the neurologist and neurosurgeon on Thursday, and surgery was on the following Tuesday. I had glioblastoma multiforme (GBM). I received radiation and chemotherapy as well as stereotactic radiation. I was very fortunate to be at a teaching hospital.

I had a recurrence in 2001 with successful resection during which they implanted Gliadel wafers.

In 2002, they thought I had another recurrence, but it was only scar tissue and radiation necrosis.

My only issues since then have been medications and a small seizure in addition to a minor impairment to my left-side peripheral vision. I continue to work full time. I know how blessed I have been, and I try to help others who are impacted by GBM and other brain tumors.

As of July 2013, things remain pretty much status quo medically.

I have learned a lot of things from my experiences; these are just a few of them:

- You will learn quickly who is comfortable and who is not comfortable in dealing with issues of mortality.
- Have someone with you to listen, ask questions, and remember. Several times the neurosurgeon told my wife that no one had ever asked him a particular question before.
- Don't fear knowledge. As my wife said many times, "There is nothing you can tell us that is worse than we can imagine."
- God gave us the gift of life that brings uncertainty. When tough times hit, He can comfort us much as we can comfort each other.

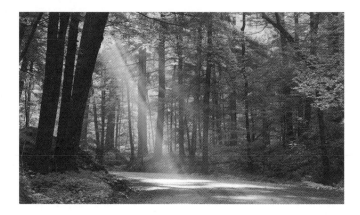

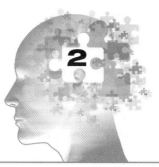

Chapter 2
From day one, a place for everything

Tools to help you get organized

The diagnosis of a brain tumor can leave patients and their loved ones in a mental fog, a fog so thick with questions that simply determining where to begin, in and of itself, can be debilitating. There are ways in which you can regain control, stepping out from the fog and into the light of day. Organization is your key to obtaining the information you'll need to find the proper treatment necessary for your specific type of tumor. The following is a list of tools that have helped other brain tumor patients.

A three-ring binder can become your best friend and treatment partner, easily safeguarding and making available at your fingertips all the necessary information about your tumor type and treatment plan. Referrals to specialists or for second or third opinions are often delayed by the need to obtain records and, sometimes, by records that have been lost along the way. Maintaining your own copies of the following items will ensure that your consulting physicians have access to all of your important documents at the time of your appointment. Many people maintain these records on their computers or flash drives and occasionally print them out and store them in the binder as needed — since it is easier to carry a binder around. Also print out a list of your current medications and allergies to store in your wallet or pocketbook in case of emergency. Items to keep in your treatment binder include:

- **Medical history.** Start with a copy of the first medical history form you are asked to fill out. This will list past medical problems, such as diabetes or heart problems, which may affect the treatment choice, as well as any allergies you have. An important allergy to note is one to either iodine or shellfish, as the dyes (contrast agents) used in some brain scans contain iodine. Having a copy of your first medical history will be helpful when you have to fill out similar forms. Keep it updated as things change. You can also ask your doctor for a copy of the history and physical examination that are performed on you.

- **Copies of MRI films and reports.** Most radiological centers today can provide you with a copy of your MRI or CT scans on a CD that can be viewed on any computer. When you check in at the MRI radiology facility, it is very important to request a copy of the film or a CD along with the written report of the radiologist's findings. Ask BEFORE you go into the scanner, as it is easier for the staff to handle the request then than if you tell them afterward. Most office supply stores carry special three-hole vinyl pages that hold multiple CDs safely within a binder.

- **All routine laboratory reports and pathology reports from biopsies.** Different members of your medical team will benefit from receiving recent laboratory results that may have been initially ordered by another physician. Having your own personal copies of all routine laboratory reports as well as **pathology reports** from biopsies, so that they are available for review on demand, will save time, increase your own understanding, and in some cases eliminate the need for unnecessary blood work. As a bonus, if you are computer literate, keep track of lab results in an Excel spreadsheet so you can graph results over time and see how you are doing.

- **Medication at a glance.** It is important to disclose *all the medications* you take to your physician and care team members. Keeping an up-to-date medication record in your treatment binder (including herbal supplements and over-the-counter items) can provide a quick and clear snapshot of your daily meds at a glance, *reducing the chance of error when more than one physician is involved with your care.* Without this information, you may experience symptoms that are medication related or side effects of a medication that one member of your medical team may not realize you are taking, with the consequence that you may be incorrectly diagnosed or treated.

Take your treatment binder to *every* appointment with *every* doctor and request that this list be reviewed before any new medication is prescribed. You should also request a copy of the drug formulary — a list of covered medications — from your insurance company and keep it in your treatment binder. It may be necessary for your physician to request prior authorization for some medications. Knowing about the need for prior authorization in advance can save you time and expense.

Pathology report (puh-THAH-loh-jee): *The description of cells and tissues made by a pathologist based on microscopic evidence and sometimes used to make a diagnosis of a disease.*

Location, location, location

Knowing the exact location of your tumor will assist you in many ways. By researching the functions of that part of the brain, you can more clearly understand — and be prepared for — many of the symptoms you are experiencing, or might expect to experience. Ask your physician to be specific about the location. Perhaps he or she can provide you with a diagram of the brain with a penciled-in identification of the tumor site. Or use the anatomical figure of the brain on the opposite page in consultation with your physician. The top part of the figure shows the major parts of the brain. The bottom part of the figure shows some of the functions associated with each of the parts.

A personal diary

Beginning on day one, keeping a diary is very important as you review various treatment options with specialists. Recording your specific questions and concerns will help ensure that your medical team provides the answers you and your loved ones or caregivers need. You may want to create a separate section for each team member, writing down which doctor is responsible for the various aspects of your care, medication refills, routine lab work, referrals, and what was discussed at appointments. Questions can often arise after you leave an appointment, and being able to refer to these pages later may be helpful. It is critical that you maintain monthly calendar pages to record the start of new medications or therapies and any bad reactions to them. The starting times of symptoms and side effects may be difficult to recall at a later date, but it is important to distinguish their origins.

Legal documents

Every doctor you see will ask you to sign a **HIPAA** privacy form. When you fill it out, write in that you want to specifically allow the following people to discuss details of your case with the doctor (or facility); then list by name your spouse / parents / children and maybe a friend. Then ask for a copy of the form, as the original will be kept by the physician in each

---

HIPAA (HIH-puh): *A 1996 US law that allows workers and their families to keep their health insurance when they change or lose their jobs. The law also includes standards for setting up secure electronic health records to protect the privacy of a person's health information and to keep it from being misused. Also called Health Insurance Portability and Accountability Act and Kassebaum Kennedy Act.*

■ Major parts of the brain

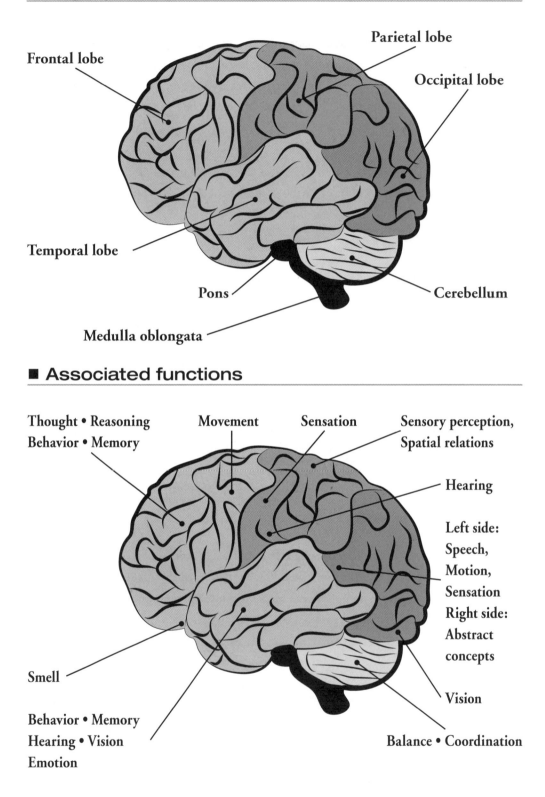

Frontal lobe

Parietal lobe

Occipital lobe

Temporal lobe

Pons

Cerebellum

Medulla oblongata

■ Associated functions

Thought • Reasoning
Behavior • Memory

Movement

Sensation

Sensory perception,
Spatial relations

Hearing

Left side:
Speech,
Motion,
Sensation
Right side:
Abstract
concepts

Smell

Vision

Behavior • Memory
Hearing • Vision
Emotion

Balance • Coordination

case. Having the copy of the executed HIPAA form will help save time when you need to send someone to pick up reports or films or to ask questions for you. When medical personnel tell you they cannot give your children something or talk about something to anyone other than you, just have the copy of the form available for them to see, and they have to meet your request.

Power-of-attorney legal documents

We all hate to think about these things, but it can save a lot of trouble later if you handle some legal matters now. An advance directive, also called a living will, tells your medical team what kind of care you would like to have if you become unable to make medical decisions. *A medical durable power of attorney* lets you designate who will make medical decisions for you if you are unable to. The first time you are admitted to a hospital, you will be asked if you want to fill out the forms for these legal documents, if you do not already have them in place. Do it, and ask for copies and keep them in your binder. Or search Google for "Advanced Directives in [your state]" (each state has different laws and forms). If you do already have these legal documents in place, bring them with you, and the staff will make copies for your files and return the originals to you.

It is very important to tell your family who your medical power of attorney will be and to tell them what your values are and what kinds of medical treatment you would want or not want, including breathing machines and feeding tubes, if your condition were to worsen and you were unable to communicate or were in a coma.

You may also want to consider drafting a *financial durable power of attorney*. A financial durable power of attorney designates a person of your choice to manage your finances if you become incapacitated and are unable to make financial decisions for yourself. Your financial power-of-attorney document should not contain medical directives, for these are covered in your medical power-of-attorney document. Standard financial durable power-of-attorney forms are available online or through an attorney. They are straightforward and easy to complete. If you have special circumstances, you may wish to consult with an attorney.

Phone numbers

Record the name, address, phone number, email address, and a short description of all of your important contacts. Be sure to include your family members who should be contacted in an emergency, all of your doctors, your lawyer, your financial advisor and/or insurance agent, and any clergy.

Second "expert" opinions

Because diagnosing a specific type of brain tumor is complicated, it is essential to get confirmation of a diagnosis. Second, third, or even fourth opinions should come from experts within a specific area, such as those who are experts in the removal of brain tumors: neurosurgeons performing at least 25 brain surgeries per year, or experts in neuropathology who can qualify the diagnosis of your tumor biopsy. It is estimated that as many as 25 percent of brain tumor patients will have their diagnosis changed upon further examination by a second, expert opinion, which can drastically change not only the **prognosis,** but also the recommended treatment plan.

If your primary brain tumor physician is not familiar with the most current treatments or clinical trials available for patients with brain tumors, request that he or she consult with one of the many major brain tumor centers and arrange for you to obtain a second expert opinion. Even if you are diagnosed by a major brain tumor center, you may still wish to get a second opinion from another major brain tumor center to confirm your diagnosis, to confirm a treatment plan, and/or to locate a clinical trial. **It is your right to have a second opinion**.

A review of your MRI or CT scans, tests, and pathology reports, along with an overview of new resources and treatment programs can be obtained through many of the leading major brain tumor centers.

Your physician can also consult with the National Cancer Institute. They will also review your case for free. They have excellent adult and pediatric brain tumor specialists available to help you.

For a list of major brain tumor treatment centers, visit: www.virtualtrials.com/btcenters.cfm.

Prognosis (prog-NO-sis): *The likely outcome or course of a disease; the chance of recovery or recurrence.*

For more information about consultations with the neuro-oncology branch (NOB) of the National Cancer Institute, select the tab for "Making Appointments," then select the tab for "Patient Referrals," after you go to: home.ccr.cancer.gov/nob/Default.aspx.

Most pathologists do not see enough brain tumors to make the subtle distinctions that may be necessary for diagnosis. You can also ask for a second opinion on the reading of the biopsy slides from a major center, such as the neuropathology division of the department of pathology at Johns Hopkins University Hospital. There is a cost, but the process is easy — your hospital just mails the slides.

For details about consultations by the division of neuropathology at Johns Hopkins University Hospital, go to: pathology.jhu.edu/department/services/consults/neuropath.cfm.

If you do need to travel for a second or third opinion, there are many organizations that provide financial assistance specifically for brain tumor patients. Please check the chapter later in this book on insurance and financial help.

The role of caregivers and loved ones

It is all too common: You enter your doctor's office with a list of questions, but as soon as your physician has finished his or her comments, you forget your own questions, or worse, forget or misunderstand the answers you receive. Emotions, not your brain tumor, are typically responsible. Emotional support and a second pair of ears can be of tremendous help while you navigate through a new world of tumor terminology.

Even for seemingly routine appointments, whenever possible, take a friend, loved one, or caregiver with you. Aside from taking notes of your session, if you become overwhelmed at any time during your physician's explanation of a particular treatment, necessary tests, or expected results, another person will be at hand to hear (or interpret) the details and will be able to ask questions that you might not think of at that moment. Encourage your companion to make frequent notations or observations in your personal treatment binder and take an active role in discussing your care options. If your physician will allow recorded sessions, have your companion manage a small hand-held recording device and review the discussion afterwards with you.

Following is a list of organizations that can help provide support for caregivers, families, and loved ones.

Support for caregivers

Cancer Care (www.cancercare.org/tagged/caregiving). This site offers stories of help and hope and has podcasts on an array of subjects ranging from financial assistance to stress management for caregivers.

Cancer Compass (www.cancercompass.com/message-board/caregivers/1,0,122.htm). This site has caregiver discussion groups and resources.

Caregiver Hope (www.caregiverhope.com). This site provides stories of hope and encouragement as cancer caregivers experience this journey starting with a loved one's diagnosis and learn to face fears, have faith and hope, and embrace life when it changes.

Caring.Com (www.caring.com). This site has articles about caregiver wellness, money, and legal matters, as well as a directory of peer-reviewed and rated home healthcare agencies, nursing homes, and hospice care.

Family Caregiver Alliance National Center on Caregiving (www.caregiver.org). This site addresses the needs of families and friends providing long-term care at home by offering national, state, and local programs to support caregivers. The site contains newsletters, fact sheets, caregiving information, and advice and online support groups.

National Hospice & Palliative Care Organization (www.nhpco.org/i4a/pages/Index.cfm?pageID=3254). This site has resources for the caregiver including preparing for caregiving, the planning-ahead checklist, caring for the caregiver, and caring for a child with a serious illness. The site also has information on advance directives.

Lotsa Helping Hands (www.lotsahelpinghands.com). This site provides an answer to the question "What can I do to help?" by allowing you to organize family and friends for needed tasks via electronic calendars and announcements. It also provides resources for caregivers.

National Family Caregivers Association (www.thefamilycaregiver.org). This site supports caregivers to those with chronic illness or disability by educating the caregiver to strive for good health and well-being. The site is a wealth of informative tips and tools for financial and medical benefits, support groups, respite care, newsletters, and publications.

Strength for Caring (www.strengthforcaring.com/index.html). This site features articles and resources just for caregivers. Share your stories and connect with other caregivers online via message boards.

Today's Caregiver (www.caregiver.com). This site offers webinars, resources, support groups, caregiver's stories, conferences, and even a book club. You can also sign up for the free Fearless Caregiver Weekly Newsletter.

Well Spouse Association (www.wellspouse.org). This site addresses the needs of caregivers with blogs, articles, and events on an array of timely pertinent subjects.

The Center to Advance Palliative Care maintains a directory of providers and resources for palliative care. To access that directory, go to: www.getpalliativecare.org.

Mind, body, soul: faith in healing and emotional wellness

While your primary physician may appear anything but spiritual in his or her approach to your brain tumor, some within the medical community are aware, and in support of, the power of prayer. Prayer, while very personal, may be empowering and proactive at times when "control" seems out of reach.

To add your name to the prayer list at the virtualtrials.com website of the Musella Foundation, go to: www.virtualtrials.com/prayer.cfm.

Also do not neglect the rest of your body. When facing a major problem like a brain tumor, the smaller problems sometimes get overlooked. You have enough problems to handle without having a "minor" problem blossom into a "major" problem. Be especially mindful of swelling and/or pain in the legs (which may indicate blood clots, unfortunately common with brain tumors), dental problems (some treatments may hurt the gums and teeth), and rashes (indicating allergic reactions to treatments).

Emotional wellness. Your life, as you once knew it, may change throughout the journey. Things may not seem normal, but there will be a new "normal" for you and your family. The new normal will be what you and your family make it. It will take time, but you will settle into a routine that is comfortable for you. As with anything that is lost, you will go through a grieving process. Although everyone experiences grief and loss differently, you will probably experience some of the universal steps in this process, which may include shock, denial, anger, depression, and acceptance.

How you work through this process will be highly personal and individual. As you work through each step, you will probably have some additional feelings that may at times present conflicts for you. These emotions are many and can be unpredictable. Neither right nor wrong, they just are, and you are entitled to feel the way you do. They may include feelings of loneliness, sorrow, anger, sadness, blame, or shame, which may lead to anxiety and stress. Sometimes you will feel helpless.

To combat such emotions, concentrate on wellness and try to work through each of the feelings rather than denying them. Have a set of coping strategies that will guide you through each step. These strategies may include: (1) accept and understand your limitations, and set realistic goals; (2) get as much up-to-date expert information about your condition as you possibly can so you don't fear the unknown, and be proactive in your treatment plan; (3) take good care of yourself by eating well, getting exercise and rest, and not self-medicating with alcohol; (4) see a mental health provider if you feel it necessary, as he or she can help you handle your emotions and stress; (5) record your feelings in a journal; and (6) try exercise, yoga, massage therapy, and/or meditation.

Palliative care can be a support mechanism for you, your caregiver, and your family. It is not new, having come on the scene for patients around the 1970s. However, today it has evolved into so much more and is provided to patients for any diagnosis, at any stage of the condition and/or treatment plan. With palliative care, you, your caregiver, and your family receive emotional support, knowledge, and resources associated with your illness to ensure that your concerns about treatment, medications, side effects, and symptoms are addressed and to enable you to make the most knowledgeable decisions about your care. The first step in seeking palliative care is to ask your doctor or cancer center. Your goals will be to reestablish the quality of your life, to ease stress, and to be more in control. It will take time and patience, but you will find your comfort zone.

At some point, you may need to transition to *hospice care,* which can be given at home, in hospitals, nursing homes, or inpatient hospice facilities. This highly specialized concept of care — given by a partnership of family members, caregivers, and medical professionals — focuses on providing ongoing comfort, emotional support, and pain management 24 hours a day. It may also include spiritual counseling for the patient and family members. Hospice care will provide medications, equipment, and any medical supplies needed, as well as physical, speech, and occupational therapies to make you feel as comfortable as possible. You will work with an interdisciplinary team including medical professionals, social workers, home health aides, clergy members, and trained volunteers. Because most people see hospice care as marking an end of life, it is often not started soon enough to provide the comfort, care, and support needed by patients, caregivers, and family members. You can always opt out of hospice care if you wish to re-enter appropriate treatment or if you experience remission. You can enter hospice care at a later time if treatments are no longer effective or if you do not wish to continue with them. Like palliative care, the main focus of hospice care is to bring quality-of-life and support services to the patient, caregivers, and family members. While palliative care may be given at any time and even through treatment, hospice care is appropriate when life expectancy is six months or less and treatments are no longer an option.

For more information about hospice care, go to the follow websites:
- The Hospice Foundation of America (www.hospicefoundation.org)
- Hospice Net (www.hospicenet.org)
- The brain-tumor help site for hospice care, Seeking Peace: Brain Tumor Hospice Care (www.brainhospice.com)

Impairments and strategies for coping

Now that you have been diagnosed with a brain tumor, you may start to experience a variety of impaired functional abilities depending on the size and location of your brain tumor and your treatment plan. You may experience depression, memory and concentration lapses, personality and mood shifts, anxiety, insomnia, difficulties with self-care, poor balance, bowel and bladder incontinence, and conversational speech and word-finding problems. Healing and recovery from surgery and treatment are very important. When you are discharged from the hospital, make sure you are given clear instructions for caring for the surgical site, for what activities you can and can't do for a period of time, for medications and dosages, and for what to do if problems develop. Arrange your ride home from the hospital and have someone at home to help you until you feel well enough to manage on your own.

Each brain reacts differently to treatment, but you can find a way to adjust and compensate. There are strategies you can use that will help you to function and feel better and in some cases regain lost functional ability.

First and foremost, speak with your medical team about your difficulties before they become more complicated. They may prescribe some medications to ease your symptoms or refer you for physical, speech, occupational, or hyperbaric therapy sessions. Physical therapists will provide exercises that strengthen your muscles, increase your flexibility and mobility, and help you regain balance. Occupational therapists will work to strengthen small muscle control and gain functionality with self-help daily activities. Speech therapists will help in developing communication skills, vocabulary, and swallowing. Neuropsychologists will help you cope with and assess cognitive and emotional changes, as well as memory, thinking skills, problem-solving and reasoning, and perception. Hyperbaric therapy sessions may be recommended to aid in healing damaged tissue. Each of the therapists may also recommend adaptive devices to help you regain some degree of functional independence.

Second, speak with your partner or family members and explain how and what you are feeling. It is important to bring people on as part of your team to support you and help make things a little easier for you. However, they need to understand what you are experiencing before they can help. The more informed they are, the better they will be able to cope, understand you, and help you set goals.

The following coping strategies have been used successfully by people in our online support group to regain quality of life. But first you must understand your strengths and weaknesses, identify or know the problems, and be willing to try a solution. At this point you may be feeling overwhelmed and confused about the changes you are experiencing. You may also feel some grief or denial for the loss of functioning. These strategies will provide the tools you and your loved ones need to help you rebuild your life.

Sometimes, the simplest solutions for what you are experiencing are organization and altering the environment. For cognitive difficulties, making notations on a legal pad, calendar, or day planner will aid memory. Include a check-off sheet or page as needed for each task completed. It will be helpful to use an alarm watch or kitchen timer to alert you of time sensitive activities. You may wish to use a weekly medicine dispenser with slots for AM and PM medications. For better concentration, you may need to minimize or avoid distractions such as loud noises. Stay focused on one task at a time or alter a task by breaking it down into smaller parts. Sometimes a daily activity or time-management chart may help organize your day. Set limits and don't schedule too many activities in one day. Rest when you need to. You may find it helpful to follow a routine by keeping a consistent schedule. Keeping daily items in predetermined designated places will make them easy to find and save time locating them.

For physical safety and comfort be aware of potential dangers in and outside of the home such as clutter, fire hazards, sharp objects, hazardous household products, scatter rugs, inadequate lighting, water heater temperature, and outside hoses. Don't forget to declutter drawers and closets. Switch to plastic cups and plates when needed. You may need to install additional handrails or place brightly colored tape across steps. You may need to conserve your energy or find it safer to use assistive aids such as canes, walkers, or wheelchairs. You may also need to install grab bars in bathroom/shower areas, use a shower seat while bathing, or purchase disposable underwear. Daily movement, which may be as simple as stretching, no matter how limited your ability, will help with improving your night's sleep, reducing negative emotions, and reducing stress, and will also help you focus.

You and your family may find it helpful to communicate with the use of word cues, picture flash cards, simple language and sentence structure, or by asking only one question at a time and repeating back information to ensure understanding. But first, make sure you are looking at the person speaking to you, so that you can focus and pick up visual cues. You may also find it helpful to play word games and puzzles.

It is important to recognize that there is no one way of doing things. You will learn to compensate for your deficits by learning new ways. Sometimes, you may feel that you have reached a plateau, but that doesn't mean that you will not progress again. You may continue to experience progress and setbacks in functioning. However, it is important to realize that when one way of doing things may no longer work for you, the strategy needs to be changed. Having patience and flexibility will be essential to your recovery. Your life will feel more normal and on track by using coping strategies that work for you. ●

KEY POINTS

☑ Get organized from day #1 with a binder to keep track of everything.

☑ Keep an up-to-date medication record in your treatment binder.

☑ Know the exact location of your tumor.

☑ Think about and execute such necessary legal documents as an advance directive, a medical durable power of attorney, and a financial durable power of attorney.

☑ Recognize that brain tumors are complicated, so second, third, and fourth opinions from experts to confirm diagnosis are essential.

☑ Whenever possible, go to all appointments with a friend, loved one, or caregiver to help you understand what physicians are saying to you.

☑ Do not neglect the rest of your body. Do not neglect your emotional health.

Survivor story #2

August 15, 2008, was a beautiful day. I was showing a retired couple a gorgeous home. They left, and I shut off the lights, locked the doors, and went out to my car. I had my hands and arms full of papers and keys, and as I was getting into my car I hit the side of my head on the top of the door frame.

I sat in the seat for a few moments, rubbing my head. After it quit hurting, I put my keys in the ignition and tried to shut my door, but it would not shut. I tried again and still it would not shut. So I looked down, and I saw that my leg was in the door, and I could not feel it or move it.

I was scared. I called 911 from my cell phone. By the time I got to the hospital, I couldn't lift my leg off the bed more than three inches. The hospital did a CT scan and said they thought I had a brain tumor but because they did not have neurological capabilities they had to transfer me to another hospital. I remember the cold, bumpy ambulance ride to the next hospital.

On August 20, I had surgery. I rolled the dice and told them to remove as much of the tumor as they could. I had a 100% tumor resection. What that means is they removed 100% of the VISIBLE tumor. The surgeon came to see me in intensive care after surgery and said it went great. The next day an oncologist came in to see me to tell me the news that I had a particularly nasty form of glioblastoma multiforme (GBM). He sent my tissue to four different laboratories to make sure he had the correct diagnosis.

I did radiation therapy and received the chemotherapeutic agent Temodar with no luck at all. In fact, I had only started the higher doses of Temodar when the tumor came back.

In February 2009, I had a second resection. Again, the neurosurgeon removed 100% of the visible tumor, and the surgeon implanted Gliadel wafers.

My oncologist started me on Irinotecan and Avastin right away. I stayed on Irinotecan for several months but eventually could not tolerate it any longer. I currently get Avastin infusions every three weeks and MRI scans every three months. As of August 2012, I am a four-year survivor. Like everyone who is a survivor, I have close friends and family who have been here for me. I could not do it without them.

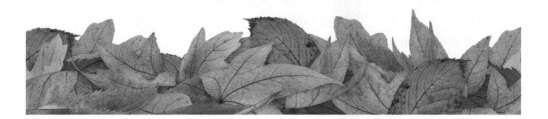

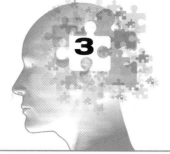

Chapter 3
Understanding brain tumors

Brain tumors are described by where they are located in the brain and what kind of cell they started from. *Primary* brain tumors originate in the brain, while *secondary* brain tumors are caused by tumor (cancer) cells that have spread to the brain from another primary source in the body, such as from breast or lung cancer.

Primary brain tumors are also classified (diagnosed), in part, by the type of cell they originate from. For example, **astrocytomas** come from astrocytes ("cyte" means cell), **oligodendrogliomas** from oligodendrocytes, **meningiomas** from meningeal cells, and **medulloblastomas** from medulloblasts ("blast" means an immature cell), just to name a few.

What is a glioma?

The most common type of primary brain tumor is a glioma, originating in the brain from glial cells. Glial cells are the "support cells" of the central nervous system, helping neurons

---

Astrocytoma (AS-troh-sy-TOH-muh): *A tumor that begins in the brain or spinal cord in small, star-shaped cells called astrocytes.*

Oligodendroglioma (AH-lih-goh-DEN-droh-glee-OH-muh): *A rare, slow-growing tumor that begins in oligodendrocytes (cells that cover and protect nerve cells in the brain and spinal cord).*

Meningioma (meh-NIN-jee-OH-muh): *A type of slow-growing tumor that forms in the meninges (thin layers of tissue that cover and protect the brain and spinal cord). Meningiomas usually occur in adults.*

Medulloblastoma (MED-yoo-loh-blas-TOH-muh): *A malignant brain tumor that begins in the lower part of the brain and that can spread to the spine or to other parts of the body.*

and nerve cells do their jobs by communicating information through electrical energy.

While glial cells can belong to several families of cells, most gliomas are made up of either astrocytes or oligodendrocytes; thus, these tumors are also frequently called astrocytomas or oligodendrogliomas (oligos). The terms glioma and astrocytoma are sometimes used interchangeably, although this is not technically correct.

High-grade (malignant) forms of these gliomas are called glioblastoma multiforme (GBM), **anaplastic** astrocytoma, and anaplastic oligodendroglioma. These gliomas are considered to be fast growing, rapidly invading nearby tissue. GBMs are the most common malignant brain tumors in adults.

Cellular makeup, speed of growth, location of the glioma, and even the age of the patient can all affect tumor behavior, resulting in a variety of symptoms and different experiences among patients. For this reason, you must guard against assuming that another person's outcome of treatment will be the same as yours.

For more information on specific types of tumors and treatments read "What You Need To Know About Brain Tumors" by the National Cancer Institute, which is located at: www.cancer.gov/cancertopics/wyntk/brain.

What does "tumor grade" mean?

All tumors are given a "grade," meaning a specific classification that relates to the current speed of growth and the potential to interfere with brain function. Grading is a determination of what stage the tumor is at, or how advanced (bad) it is in its development.

Grading a specific tumor type has been described as something that is as much an "art form" as a science and is typically a determination made by a pathologist after a biopsy. Grading can be somewhat controversial depending on the size of biopsy specimen obtained. One part of the tumor may have smaller lower-grade cells, while larger more aggressive cells may be present in a different location in the tumor. Furthermore, tumors initially assigned a low grade can become aggressive in growth, changing the status of the grade even during the course of treatment. It is important to have your biopsy examined by a neuropathologist who sees a large number of brain tumors, always requesting a copy of the report for your records and comparison.

Anaplastic (A-nuh-PLAS-tik): *A term used to describe cancer cells that divide rapidly and have little or no resemblance to normal cells.*

Both the type and the grade of a tumor are critical for your diagnosis and treatment. That is why getting a second opinion regarding biopsy specimens is so important.

The most common grading system is called the WHO system, based on its approval by the World Health Organization. The WHO system classifies all cancers on a grade of I to IV (1 to 4). A grade of I or II designates slow-growing "benign" tumors, while a grade of III or IV designates faster growing tumors that are considered malignant. A grade III tumor is called an anaplastic astrocytoma, and a grade IV tumor is called GBM.

When dealing with brain tumors, the word "benign" is a little misleading. It implies that the tumor is not dangerous. Because the brain is enclosed in a rigid container (the skull), there is no space for a tumor mass to grow. As a tumor (even a "benign" tumor) grows, it builds up intracranial pressure and compresses everything around it, which can lead to neurological problems and even death. Luckily, there has been a lot of progress in the treatment of benign brain tumors. One type of benign tumor, the acoustic neuroma, used to be incurable and fatal. Now it can be cured in over 95% of patients, sometimes with a relatively simple radiation procedure. There is controversy over which way to treat an acoustic neuroma, either by radiation or surgery, but both options are so good that the decision is now made by trying to determine which treatment will have fewer side effects, as both may be curative.

Just be aware that a few hospitals employ a different grading system for brain tumors, using a scale of grades 1 to 3, with WHO grades I and II combined into "grade 1" and with the rest of the WHO grades moved down a grade: an anaplastic astrocytoma is thus a grade 2, and a GBM is thus a grade 3. The terms anaplastic astrocytoma and GBM are more precise.

How long has the tumor been there?

Nobody really knows how long you have had your particular tumor. Slow-growing tumors can be present for years without causing any symptoms. Fast-growing tumors can occur and cause symptoms within a span of six months or less.

Are brain tumors the same as brain cancer?

This question is controversial. There are arguments for both sides. Some people argue that because a brain tumor rarely spreads outside the brain, it cannot be considered a cancer. Other people argue that because a brain tumor has the potential to grow and be deadly, it should be considered a cancer. We feel that brain tumors are cancers.

Can brain tumors be removed surgically?

In many cases, brain tumors can be removed by surgery. Surgery may actually "cure" some low-grade tumors, such as acoustic neuroma. However, for high-grade tumors, surgery is not a cure, but it does buy time for other treatments to work, and it offers a lot of opportunities. For example, a tissue sample from surgery can be used for biopsy and can undergo testing for drug resistance. Moreover, there are some therapies that require prior surgery and removal of the tumor. One such important therapy is the **Gliadel wafer,** a dissolvable wafer impregnated with a chemotherapeutic agent that is directly implanted at the site of tumor removal. Another is **brachytherapy** by means of the Gliasite Radiation Therapy System — an internal radiation therapy that requires placing radioactive material directly at the tumor site.

3

Any tumor can theoretically be removed, but the neurosurgeon uses his or her experience to make a judgment on the risks of removal versus the benefits of removal. Each brain tumor is different, but the neurosurgeon can usually predict if — and how much — neurological damage will occur if the brain tumor is removed. Since surgery of high-grade brain tumors is not a cure, sometimes brain tumors are considered inoperable if the expected neurological damage arising from the surgery would create unacceptable problems for the patient.

In brain surgery, experience matters A LOT. Neurosurgeons who have operated on a lot of tumors can usually remove more of the tumor, with fewer side effects, than neurosurgeons who have operated only on a few tumors. They are also much more likely to have the latest high-tech surgical tools available. In general, the more of the tumor removed, the better the outcome. That is why one of the single most important decisions you have to make is WHERE and by WHOM you will have brain surgery. A more experienced neurosurgeon may consider relatively easy what another neurosurgeon might consider inoperable.

However, keep in mind that some neurosurgeons may be overly aggressive. Discuss the expected risks of the surgery to make sure your neurosurgeon understands your views on how aggressive you want him or her to be.

Gliadel wafer (GLY-uh-del WAY-fer): *A biodegradable wafer that is used to deliver the anticancer drug carmustine directly into a brain tumor site after the tumor has been removed by surgery. Also called polifeprosan 20 carmustine implant.*

Brachytherapy (BRAY-kee-THAYR-uh-pee): *A type of radiation therapy in which radioactive material sealed in needles, seeds, wires, or catheters is placed directly into or near a tumor. Also called implant radiation therapy, internal radiation therapy, and radiation brachytherapy.*

Furthermore, while there are over 4500 neurosurgeons in the United States, only 125 (approximately) are considered experts in the removal of brain tumors, performing these delicate surgeries at least 25 times per year or more. Again, because choosing an experienced neurosurgeon can greatly affect the quality of tumor removal and your recovery, getting a second opinion about which neurosurgeon to choose is vital.

What are the survival statistics for patients with brain tumors?

Nobody knows how long you are going to live with your brain tumor. Statistics are a tool used for comparing treatments and for describing what has happened in the past to groups of people with your tumor type. *They cannot predict how long any individual person will live.*

There are two important survival statistics that you will commonly see in research about brain tumors: *overall survival (OS)* and *progression-free survival (PFS)*. OS is the percentage of people in the group under study who are alive at a certain point in time — such as 1 or 2 years. Just because a 1-year or 2-year survival statistic is reported does not mean that you will live for 1 or 2 years. Rather, it means that on average the people described in that particular research lived for that length of time.

PFS is reported either as the percentage of people who reach a milestone without having tumor progression — such as 6 months or 1 year — or as the average number of months before tumor progression for the entire group. Progression means tumor recurrence. The survival statistics of OS and PFS are commonly used in medical research, and you can compare treatments by looking at either number. We feel that PFS is the more important survival statistic because after people experience tumor progression, they usually move on to other treatments. In that case, relying on the OS survival statistic to evaluate a treatment may be misleading.

As you read about survival statistics, keep in mind that they fail to take into consideration many factors that are extremely important on a case-by-case patient basis — such as age, general health, tumor size and location within the brain, the extent of tumor removal by neurosurgery, and much more, including access to the care of brain tumor experts.

Surgical technologies and the ability to accurately diagnose brain tumors have improved dramatically, and ongoing clinical trials are leading the way to new and better treatments. Your ability to challenge survival statistics will greatly depend on surrounding yourself with a medical team that is not influenced negatively by such numbers.

Try to avoid those within the medical community who have an unfortunate and bleak outlook and may not be current in their understanding of progressive new treatments. Physicians associated with, and in consultation with, leading brain tumor medical centers are your best defense against negative survival statistics and will enhance your ability to remain positively engaged during your journey through treatment.

The well-known evolutionary biologist and Harvard University professor Stephen J. Gould wrote something of a guide to surviving survival statistics after his diagnosis with a rare abdominal tumor called mesothelioma. His famous 1985 essay "The Median Isn't the Message" can be found at Steve Dunn's cancer guide at <u>cancerguide.org/median_not_msg.html</u>.

Look for people with your tumor type who are leading normal lives. These people prove that no tumor type is completely hopeless. Participate in online and real-world support groups, discussed later in this book, to meet others who have gone through the same medical crisis as you but are now many years out and doing well. It is important to see and acknowlege that there are people with brain tumors who do well. ●

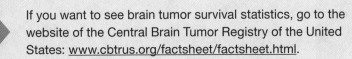

If you want to see brain tumor survival statistics, go to the website of the Central Brain Tumor Registry of the United States: <u>www.cbtrus.org/factsheet/factsheet.html</u>.

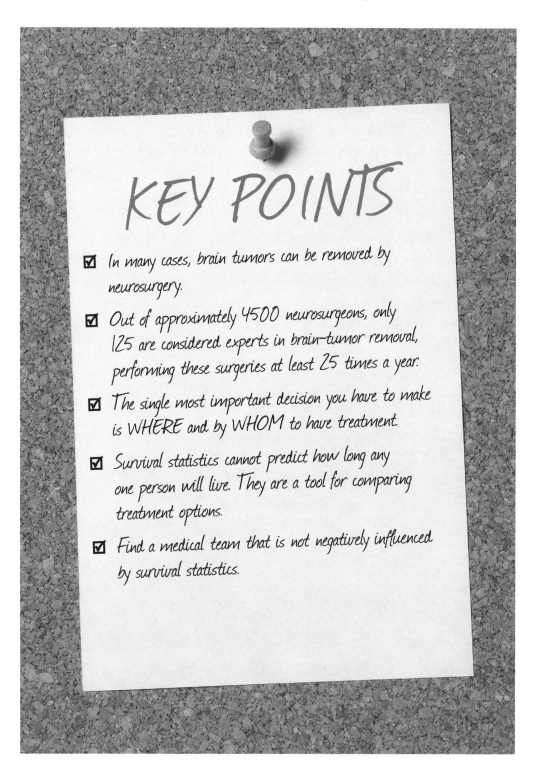

KEY POINTS

☑ In many cases, brain tumors can be removed by neurosurgery.

☑ Out of approximately 4500 neurosurgeons, only 125 are considered experts in brain-tumor removal, performing these surgeries at least 25 times a year.

☑ The single most important decision you have to make is WHERE and by WHOM to have treatment.

☑ Survival statistics cannot predict how long any one person will live. They are a tool for comparing treatment options.

☑ Find a medical team that is not negatively influenced by survival statistics.

Survivor story #3

On April 9, 2008, when I was 43 years old, my world changed. A few hours after a long transatlantic flight, green lights suddenly started to appear in front of me. First two, then four, then eight green lights. When I came to, I saw my wife and sister hugging each other and in tears. Witnessing a grand mal seizure was probably the most frightening thing they had ever seen. I was transported by ambulance to the local emergency room, and a subsequent CT scan showed a lesion in my left temporal lobe. In this way, a brain tumor introduced itself into our lives.

Three weeks later, I was lucky to be connected to a surgeon with a "let's take this tumor on!" attitude. After an aggressive but successful surgery, he removed all "visible" tumor from my left temporal lobe. Pathology showed that I had glioblastoma multiforme (GBM) with oligodendrocytes. I wound up going under the knife a second time, two weeks later, because of an infection.

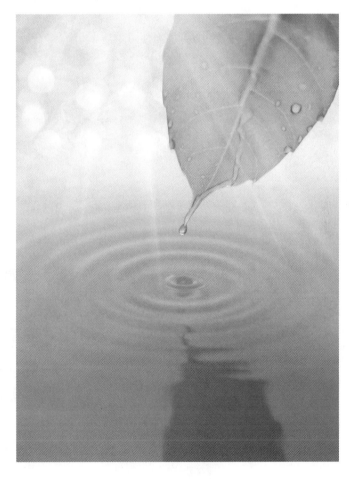

Radiation therapy started in June 2008 for six weeks. Chemotherapy with Temodar also started on a 5-day-on, 23-day-off monthly cycle and then became bimonthly. I continue to receive MRI scans every two to three months.

After surgery, I was unable to talk for several months. I could not read or write for about a year. I still have some difficulty.

From early on, I got support from our local wellness community — free mindfulness meditation and yoga classes. I try to keep stress to a minimum.

I work with a nutritionist who helps me try to stay on track with eating right and maintaining a healthy internal terrain.

It is now four years and four months since my diagnosis. Who knows why I've been so lucky. Attitude? Love? Eating right? Exercise? Surgery + radiation + chemotherapy? All the other things I do? I just don't know. But I do know that I am grateful for today, and that I couldn't have made it this far without immense help from friends, family, doctors, nurses, and above all my wife.

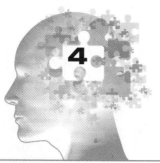

Chapter 4
Your medical team, questions to ask, and brain scans

Your medical team will include several experts experienced in different medical specialties. These different specialties might be neuro-oncology (the medical treatment of brain tumors), neurology (conditions of the nervous system, such as the brain and spinal cord), surgery, radiology (MRI/CT), **radiation therapy,** and pathology (the study of tissue). The make-up of your medical team will vary depending on the type and location of your tumor, and it may include experts representing a variety of different medical cross-specialties. It is essential that your medical team include experts experienced *specifically in the treatment of brain tumors.*

A medical (board-certified) oncologist treats many forms of cancer; however, not all oncologists are experts in treating brain tumors. As part of your medical team, your general oncologist can assist you with obtaining second opinions and researching available treatment options, but he or she should refer you to a neuro-oncologist experienced specifically in the treatment of brain tumors. Most neuro-oncologists are also neurologists, treating disorders of the nervous system (some also started as general oncologists) as well as general cancer. It is important that you establish that he or she is experienced in treating your type of tumor and is up-to-date on advances in both surgery and alternative treatments. If a neuro-oncologist is not available in your area, an experienced oncologist is the next best thing.

Radiation therapy (RAY-dee-AY-shun THAYR-uh-pee): *The use of high-energy radiation from x-rays, gamma rays, neutrons, protons, and other sources to kill cancer cells and shrink tumors. Radiation may come from a machine outside the body (external-beam radiation therapy), or it may come from radioactive material placed in the body near cancer cells (internal radiation therapy).*

A *neurosurgeon* is someone who performs surgery involving the nervous system, typically specializing in one particular area or system, such as the spine. Before considering any surgical procedure, it is important to know the experience level of your neurosurgeon, opting for a second opinion (preferably) from a neurosurgeon associated with a major brain tumor center. While some neurosurgeons also practice neuro-oncology and oversee the administration of chemotherapy treatments, most confine their practice to surgical therapy and follow-up care.

A *neuro-radiologist* is a specialist in the area of reading MRI and CT scans involving the nervous system. Your MRI or CT scans should always be reviewed by a neuro-radiologist experienced with tumors within the brain.

A *radiation oncologist* specializes in the administration of radiation therapy (solely and specifically) and should work in cooperation with your neuro-oncologist/surgeon to develop an appropriate course for the duration and intensity of your radiation therapy.

You should consider other specialists for complementary care throughout your treatment and recovery, such as:

- Rehabilitation specialists (physical/speech therapist, occupational therapist)
- Neuropsychologists and psychiatrists
- **Endocrinologists**
- Ophthalmologists (eye doctors)
- Dentists (especially important prior to chemotherapy)
- Pharmacists
- Nutritionists
- The group of doctors at your hospital of care who might undertake the **tumor board review** of your tumor treatment

---

Endocrinologist (en-doh-krih-NAH-loh-jist): *A doctor who specializes in the diagnosis and treatment of disorders of the endocrine system (the glands and organs that make hormones). These disorders include diabetes, infertility, and thyroid, adrenal, and pituitary gland problems.*

Tumor board review (TOO-mer bord reh-VYOO): *A treatment planning approach in which a number of doctors who are experts in different specialties (disciplines) review and discuss the medical condition and treatment options of a patient. In cancer treatment, a tumor board review may include that of a medical oncologist (who provides cancer treatment with drugs), a surgical oncologist (who provides cancer treatment with surgery), and a radiation oncologist (who provides cancer treatment with radiation). Also called multidisciplinary opinion.*

What questions should I ask my medical team?

- What type of brain cancer do I have?
- What is the grade of the brain cancer?
- Are any additional tests needed?
- How many tumor types like this do you treat each year?
- Will the brain tumor board review my case? How often?
- Where would you recommend I get a confirming/second opinion?
- Do you have any written information about my type of brain cancer?
- How will the brain tumor affect my functioning?
- What are my treatment options?
- Which treatment do you recommend? Why?
- Which clinical trials do I qualify for, and which do you recommend?
- Can you recommend an oncologist who specializes in this type of brain cancer?
- What other specialists will be part of my care?
- What is the timeline for treatment(s)?
- Where will I get the treatment?
- Will I be able to drive myself to and from treatment?
- Will my medical insurance cover this type of treatment?
- How will this type of treatment affect my work schedule?
- Will I need to apply for disability? Social security disability?
- Will I need to take medications? If so, what kinds and how often?
- Are there any side effects? What kind?
- Are there short-term and long-term side effects?
- How can side effects be managed? By medicines? By physical therapy?
- Will my quality of life change? Will I function differently?
- Will I see a change in my personality? Appetite? Sleep habits? Memory?
- What can I expect before, during, and after treatment?
- What is the follow-up plan if this treatment doesn't work?
- How often will I need follow-up imaging scans? What kind of scans?
- Do you think I should attend a support group now? Are there any support groups nearby?

All about brain scans

Brain scans allow the doctors to get an idea of what is going on inside the head. No scan is 100% accurate, and each is open to interpretation. The more experienced the doctor is at interpreting brain scans, the more confident you can be about the results of that interpretation. As mentioned elsewhere, it is a good idea to get a personal copy of the films (or a CD of them) and the radiology report. You can share these documents with your medical team to make sure they agree on the reading of the scans. Having copies of the scans will also be useful if you need a quick second opinion from another brain tumor center, as well as in case the original scans are lost, which happens more than you would think!

A *CT scan* (or CAT scan, a computerized axial tomogram) uses x-rays to generate a computer simulation picture of the cross section of your head. Usually, a contrast agent (a dye) is injected into your arm halfway through the test to enable the tumor to show up better. A CT scan can be readily available and much cheaper than an MRI scan. A CT scan shows some things very well, such as bleeding into the brain and signs of swelling, and it is sometimes used for planning surgery and radiation. Since CT scans use x-rays, there is a tiny risk with their use, so they are usually limited to only when they are absolutely needed, especially in children. If you are having a CT scan performed on a child, ask the radiology technician whether the level of exposure dosage can be reduced appropriately for children. On some older CT scanners, such a reduction is not possible, and you should select a different imaging facility.

An *MRI scan* (magnetic resonance imaging) uses magnetism and radio waves to create a "picture" of the inside of your head. It is more detailed than a CT scan and usually preferred when trying to diagnose a brain tumor. An MRI scan will find smaller tumors than a CT scan. A different contrast agent is used for MRI scans than for CT scans, so if you had an allergic reaction to the dye used for a CT scan, you can still usually use the contrast agent for an MRI scan (and vice versa). Sometimes you cannot have a MRI scan if there is any metal in your body. If there is any metal in your body, mention that when you make the appointment so they can determine whether the scanning is safe. Other than the problem with metal, and a small risk with the contrast agent, MRI scans are thought to be safe.

There are many available kinds of MRI scans. Here are some of the important ones:

- **MRA** (magnetic resonance angiography) shows details of the blood vessels.

- **MRS** (magnetic resonance spectroscopy) shows the chemical makeup of the brain, which can sometimes be used to tell the difference between radiation necrosis, normal brain, swelling, and tumor. Sometimes, MRS can distinguish between low-grade and high-grade tumors, which is helpful when picking the best area for a biopsy. MRS is much faster than regular MRI for determining if treatments are working, and it is most useful when repeated to compare with the previous scan to see if you are getting better or worse. MRS is available at most brain tumor centers and is starting to become available everywhere.

- **fMRI** (functional MRI) measures blood flow in the brain and is used to map which areas of your brain control which functions. For example, if the tumor is near your speech area, you will be asked to talk while the scan is performed to highlight the areas you use while talking, and to see if the tumor invades that area.

- **Diffusion MRI** measures water movement in the brain. It can be used to determine how well the treatment is working.

- **PET** (positron emission tomography) uses a tiny amount of a radioactive substance injected into your arm. PET shows how metabolically active each area of the brain is based on how much glucose is being used. Differences in metabolic activity can help distinguish normal brain from areas affected by a brain tumor. The use of PET scans is not available everywhere, and it is expensive. ●

For breaking news about brain tumor treatments, visit regularly the news page of the Musella Foundation website, virtualtrials.com, and subscribe to the brain tumor news blast. Go to: www.virtualtrials.com/news.cfm.

KEY POINTS

☑ Understand the different functions of the members of your medical treatment team.

☑ Make yourself certain that the members of your medical team are experienced specifically in the treatment of brain tumors.

☑ Using the questions here as a guide, prepare a list of questions, and be sure to ask the members of your medical treatment team about treatment options.

☑ Get copies of your brain scans (or a CD of them) and their interpretations, and share them with and show them to other members of your medical team to ensure that they agree with the interpretations.

Survivor story #4

I am a 44-year-old woman who was diagnosed with oligodendroglioma on Christmas Day in 2006. Since the original surgical resection of the tumor, my low-grade glioma has gradually recurred over time, and I have undergone various other treatments, including a vaccine clinical trial and a chemotherapeutic course with Temodar.

For the past 4 months, I have been using Optune, and I want to share my positive experience with the device. I have heard that some people might be reluctant to use it because of the way it looks or because they feel that it will compromise their quality of life. These have been non-issues for me.

I am a fit, athletic woman who has done some modeling. If anyone would be concerned about her appearance, it would be me.

But it never entered my mind not to use Optune because I would need to shave my head. It is easy to conceal the Optune arrays with a hat, head scarf, or wig. Wigs today are high quality and so realistic that it is often impossible to tell when a person is wearing one. In addition, once a year the American Cancer Society offers a free wig made of real hair to women in cancer treatment — as well as free hats and scarves.

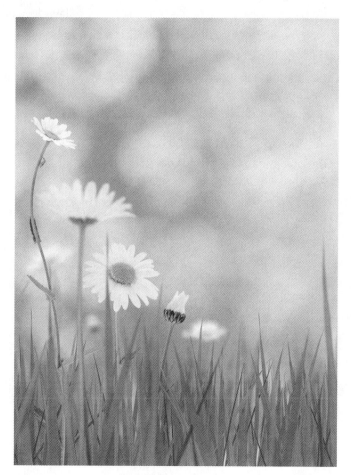

The accompanying battery for the Optune device is carried in a bag that goes over the shoulder or can be worn as a backpack. The bag no more encumbers me than a purse. If you can carry a purse or briefcase, you can carry the Optune bag.

I work as a librarian in a public library, dealing with the public all day. Most people do not notice that I am different in any way, and I get a lot of compliments on my head scarves. At the reference desk, I place the Optune battery bag next to my chair with the strap over my shoulder. The bag is not only unnoticeable but ready to go if I need to stand up and walk. The cord runs from the back of my head down my back under my shirt, connecting to the battery in the bag.

The reason to use Optune is that it does not compromise one's lifestyle or well-being as other treatments can do. I have been through debilitating chemotherapy treatments, and I have dealt with nausea, low blood counts, and fatigue. I have also been through a clinical trial that took place across the country, and for a period of 18 months, I had to leave my family and job to travel every 3 weeks to the trial site. That had a huge negative impact on my quality of life. With Optune, I am able to hike for miles, ride a bike, shovel snow, play with my dogs, and attend my children's music concerts, plays, cross-country meets, and ski races — anything and everything I would do if I were not wearing it.

The only issue for many users of Optune is skin irritation caused by having the skin covered by the electrodes for long periods of time. The irritation can be easily managed by changing the Optune electrodes every few days and, when doing so, taking some time off from treatment to allow the skin to breathe. During that time, I do the two things I can't otherwise do while wearing the device — swimming and running. Other than during these electrode changes, I wear the device 24 hours a day.

Optune is the first major advance in brain tumor treatment in a decade. It is a fantastic non-toxic, non-invasive, non-damaging, non-clinical-trial-disqualifying treatment. I am thrilled to have the opportunity to use it before I might have to deal with neurological damage from the tumor that could leave me disabled and cognitively impaired.

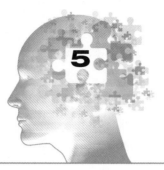

Chapter 5
Treatments of brain tumors

Surgery is usually the first treatment for a brain tumor. For some low-grade brain tumors, surgery can be curative, and no further treatment will be needed. Unfortunately, for the majority of brain tumors, even though surgery is successful, additional treatments are needed. That is because surgery by itself, even with the most advanced surgical techniques, is unable to remove all the cancer cells.

Because it is not possible to remove all the cancer cells by means of surgery, even before surgery takes place you need to be preparing with your medical team a list of options for postsurgical treatment. Here are some of the things you should request and/ or ask about even before surgery occurs.

- Before surgery, request genetic testing of your tumor tissue. There are genetic markers in tumors that can indicate drug resistance and thus influence choices about postsurgical treatment. In addition, specific genetic mutations can determine eligibility for specifically targeted immunotherapy trials or for drugs that are approved for types of cancer other than brain tumors. Major brain tumor centers routinely perform genetic testing of tumors, but you should ask anyway. Companies that can perform a complete genetic and mutational testing of your tumor are Caris Life Sciences (www.carislifesciences.com) and Foundation Medicine (www.foundationmedicine.com). Although this service is expensive, some insurance companies cover the expense.

- Before surgery, find out how your brain tumor tissue will be preserved after extraction. If the specimen will not be immediately used either to create a custom-made vaccine or to serve for genetic testing, ask if the specimen can be frozen for future use if needed, and ask about the costs involved.

- Before surgery, ask about personalized vaccine therapy, which requires a tumor sample.

- Before surgery, ask about clinical trials that require registration even before surgery occurs.

- Before surgery, ask about the possibility of implantation of Gliadel wafers within the brain tumor cavity during surgery. The chemotherapeutic drug contained in the dissolvable Gliadel wafers can begin treating residual cancer cells even before post-surgical radiation therapy and systemic chemotherapy begin. Be aware that implantation of Gliadel wafers during surgery may make you ineligible for some clinical trials, and plan ahead.

Be aware that most long-term survivors of high-grade glioma have had multiple surgeries. Usually, surgery will not be as bad as you expect. The worst part may just be worrying about it the night before. There are risks to surgery anywhere in the body, but surgery today is much safer and easier than it was even 10 years ago. Serious side effects are much less common than they used to be, so don't let horror stories from the past bother you. Problems still do occur but not as frequently as in the past.

Standard-of-care treatment for high-grade glioma

The current standard-of-care treatment for newly diagnosed high-grade malignant glioma consists of a combination of up to 5 different treatments, depending on patient and tumor characteristics: (1) surgery; (2) implantation of Gliadel wafers in the tumor cavity during surgery; (3) radiation therapy; (4) oral chemotherapy during and after radiotherapy; and (5) alternating electric field therapy (the Optune device) after radiotherapy. In the pages that follow, these different treatments are described.

Radiation therapy starts a few weeks after surgery and takes place 5 days per week for 6 weeks. Concomitant treatment with the chemotherapeutic agent **Temodar** (the generic name is temozolomide) starts at the same time as radiation therapy. After the 6-week course of radiation therapy and Temodar is completed, treatment with Temodar continues (referred to as "adjuvant therapy" from that point forward). For patients with

---

Temodar (TEH-moh-dar): *A drug that is used to treat certain types of brain tumors in adults and is being studied in the treatment of other types of cancer. It belongs to the family of drugs called alkylating agents.*

The National Comprehensive Cancer Network (NCCN) is a not-for-profit alliance of 27 of the leading cancer centers in the United States. The NCCN publishes evidence-based, consensus-driven guidelines for the treatment of different types of cancers, including guidelines for the treatment of brain tumors in the document entitled "Central Nervous System Cancers." The standard-of-care treatment for high-grade glioma that is described in this book comes from the most recent version of this guideline, dated July 25, 2016. To access this guideline, go to: www.nccn.org/professionals/physician_gls/pdf/cns.pdf. You may have to register before downloading the guideline.

glioblastoma multiforme (GBM), Temodar is approved by the FDA for six 28-day cycles of adjuvant therapy, with the drug administered on days 1 to 5 of each 28-day cycle. Currently, it is not known how long Temodar should be administered. Some doctors use Temodar for a specific time period, such as 12, 18, or 24 months, while others use it until it stops working or causes side effects or until the tumor is either completely gone or sufficiently stable. During the adjuvant Temodar stage, alternating electric field therapy with the Optune device can take place.

If this standard-of-care treatment is not offered to you, you should ask why not. If cost is the barrier to receiving this treatment, contact us. The Musella Foundation has a co-payment assistance program that may be able to help you in some circumstances with your out-of-pocket expenses.

In some cases, if there is still tumor on the scan after standard radiation therapy, an additional dose of a much-focused form of radiation, called **stereotactic radiotherapy**, may be tried. Stereotactic radiotherapy is described below. If these treatments do not work, then other therapies are considered.

Stereotactic radiotherapy (STAYR-ee-oh-TAK-tik RAY-dee-oh-THAYR-uh-pee):
A type of external radiation therapy that uses special equipment to position the patient and precisely give a single large dose of radiation to a tumor. It is used to treat brain tumors and other brain disorders that cannot be treated by regular surgery. It is also being studied in the treatment of other types of cancer. Also called radiation surgery, radiosurgery, and stereotaxic radiosurgery.

Treatments and the Food and Drug Administration

There are two general classes of treatment: (1) those approved by the FDA specifically for brain tumors on the basis of evidence from clinical trials; and (2) experimental treatments, sometimes with drugs approved by the FDA for other types of cancers or other diseases, and sometimes with drugs not yet approved at all by the FDA.

Currently, there are only a few drugs approved by the FDA specifically for the treatment of brain tumors. More than 30 years ago, the alkylating chemotherapeutic agents BCNU and CCNU were approved for "brain tumors." More recently, for the FDA indication of "newly diagnosed high-grade gliomas," the Gliadel wafer (biodegradable wafers impregnated with BCNU) and Temodar have been approved. Similarly, for the precise FDA indication of "recurrent glioblastoma multiforme," the Gliadel wafer and **Avastin** have been approved.

Even if an FDA-approved drug is not approved specifically for "brain tumors," your medical team is still able to prescribe it for your brain tumor. When doctors prescribe a drug for a therapeutic purpose other than the one approved by the FDA, it is called "off-label" prescribing. Many drugs commonly used for brain tumors are used off label. Although the use of these drugs by your medical team is legal, and the drugs are easily available, you might nonetheless have trouble getting your insurance company to pay for a drug's off-label usage because it will argue that such off-label treatment is experimental. In such cases, know that you can fight the insurance company's denial. You should enlist your neuro-oncologist to help get the drug approved by your insurance company.

A clinical trial (defined below) is the best way of trying experimental therapies, for the doctors will watch you very carefully for signs of side effects. Be aware that there is a mechanism for using an experimental drug outside of clinical trials, but it is only for those who do not qualify for the usually rigid entrance criteria of clinical trials. This mechanism is called "compassionate usage." People in clinical trials seem to do better than people who choose not to participate. This may be due to the fact that you are watched more closely while in a trial than when not in a trial. Also, once a cure is actually found, the first people

---

Avastin (uh-VAS-tin): *A drug used to treat glioblastoma (a type of brain cancer) and certain types of colorectal cancer, lung cancer, and kidney cancer. It is also being studied in the treatment of other types of cancer. Avastin binds to a protein called vascular endothelial growth factor (VEGF). This may prevent the growth of new blood vessels that tumors need to grow. It is a type of antiangiogenesis agent and a type of monoclonal antibody. Also called bevacizumab.*

to get it will be those in the clinical trial for it. Cures have been found for other types of cancer, and it will happen for brain tumors, hopefully someday soon.

Clinical trials

Clinical trials offer experimental treatments that may provide new inroads to extended life expectancy and an improved quality of life. Understanding the current availability of clinical trials requires time and due diligence. We hate to say this, but some doctors are reluctant to refer you to other treatment centers. You must search out for yourself the appropriate clinical trials available for your specific tumor-type, always advocating in your own best interests toward a cure.

Understanding clinical trials

Most clinical trials are designated as phase I, II, or III trials, a designation based upon specific questions that a particular study is seeking to answer. These clinical trial phases are defined by the FDA in the ***Code of Federal Regulations.***

- **In phase I trials,** a new drug or treatment is studied in a small group of people (20 to 80 patients or volunteers) for the first time to evaluate its safety, determine a safe dosage range, and identify potential side effects.

- **In phase II trials,** the study drug or treatment is given to a larger group of people (100 to 300 patients) and further measured for effectiveness and safety. Dosage of medication may be increased to determine toxicity levels.

- **In phase III trials,** the study drug or treatment is given to large groups of people (300 to 3000 patients) to confirm its effectiveness within a sizable population, monitor side effects and toxicity levels, compare it with standard treatments, and further determine safety.

Why should I consider participating in a clinical trial?

Clinical trials provide access to some of the newest and most promising treatments for diseases that have no cure. In many cases, these trials, guided by experts, may represent your best possible chance for survival or for a better quality of life. By participating in a clinical trial, you help researchers take one small step, or even a giant leap, closer to a cure. Aside from helping yourself, your experiences help advance the state of the art in the field, which may lead to better treatments in the future.

Another advantage to enrolling in a clinical trial is the cost. All brain tumor treatments are very expensive. In general, the experimental treatment used in a clinical trial is free to you. There may, however, be charges for associated costs of treatment — such as surgery, doctor's consultations and visits, MRI scans, blood tests, and others — so ask about costs and what your insurance will pay and what your out-of-pocket expenses will be. If you have no insurance, there may be clinical trials available that cover all the costs.

When should I consider a clinical trial?

The decision of when to participate in a clinical trial should be discussed with your medical team. Some patients and physicians feel more comfortable exhausting traditional treatment avenues first. Others choose to participate in trials from the onset of diagnosis. You may wish to discuss certain points of progress (or lack of progress) with your medical team as a guideline to help you with your decision. Obviously, if you have a low-grade tumor for which good treatments are available, you will be less likely to try something experimental. If you have a high-grade tumor and the expected outcome of the standard treatments is not acceptable to you, it is easier to make the decision to try something experimental.

Clinical trials have their own sets of eligibility requirements that might include the age range of participants, location of the tumor, grade and/or type of tumor, or the specific degree of stabilization before admission into the trial. Some clinical trials are specific for treatment of recurring tumors rather than treatment of newly diagnosed tumors. Whether or not you decide to wait or move forward, it is important to research available trials early for your specific type of tumor and know in advance if, or when, you might qualify. Be especially careful not to miss trial-entry deadlines. Some trials require that you sign up for them *before surgery*. Others require that you sign up before radiation therapy ends.

One thing to keep in mind is to plan ahead and think through a large range of contingencies. Some types of treatments might disqualify you from later trying some experimental treatments. In such a case, you will usually not have enough real data to make an informed decision. In the old days, it was an easy decision — the standard-of-care treatment provided so little hope that you had nothing to lose. But the current standard-of-care treatment has progressed to the point where you now have a difficult decision to make about when to enter a clinical trial, as the standard-of-care treatment does help some people for a long time.

How do I assess a clinical trial?

The best way to evaluate if a clinical trial is right for you is to speak with your primary physician, your neuro-oncologist or surgeon, and other members of your medical team, including those to whom you have turned for second opinions. You might also contact one of the major brain tumor centers for additional insight into a specific clinical trial. You should also consult with the physician in charge of the trial. It is always helpful to know how earlier trials of the proposed treatment came out. Lastly, it is important to ask any physicians not in favor of your participation: Why not? What would they recommend instead, and why?

Although individual cases are meaningless statistically, the experiences of others may help give you enough information to choose between two treatments that are otherwise a toss-up. You can find these individual experiences in the online support groups, real-world support groups, and in the results of the Brain Tumor Virtual Trial, a study run by the Musella Foundation (see below).

How do I find clinical trials?

You can find listings for clinical trials at the virtualtrials.com website of the Musella Foundation, at the National Cancer Institute website, and at the registry of clinical trials run by the US National Institutes of Health and called clinicaltrials.gov.

- At the virtualtrials.com website of the Musella Foundation, under the tab "Find a Treatment," clinical trials can be sorted in multiple ways: by country, by state, by tumor type, by the date the clinical trial was listed, and by the number of partici-pating centers. You can also use key words — such as a name of a cancer center or the name of a doctor — to search for specific clinical trials. The Musella Foundation can also be directly called at 1-888-295-4740. To access the "Find a Treatment" tab, go to: www.virtualtrials.com.

- The National Cancer Institute is not specific to brain tumors, but it does maintain a powerful clinical-trials search engine. In addition to allowing you to search by cancer type, location, and other variables, it also allows you to search by the type of trial (that is, whether it is a phase I, phase II, or phase III trial). To access the National Cancer Institute clinical-trial-search engine, go to: www.cancer.gov/clinicaltrials/search.

- Clinicaltrials.gov is the world's largest clinical trials database, currently holding registrations from over 130,000 trials from more than 170 countries. You can search for trials by condition, intervention, sponsor, location, and type of trial. To access clinicaltrials.gov, go to: www.clinicaltrials.gov.

Neurosurgery

Surgery is performed to improve neurological function, to confirm your diagnosis by means of a biopsy ("open biopsy" or "stereotactic biopsy"), or to completely ("total resection") or partially ("sub-total resection" or "**debulking**") remove the tumor. With a resection, you should get a biopsy of the sample removed. You should ask your surgeon for a copy of the pathology report. You can easily (but it may be expensive — check first) get a second opinion on the reading of the pathology slides. There is a lot of interpretation put into the reading of the slides, and **this is the single most important test you will ever have in your life**, so it may be worth the money to double-check it. Best of all, getting a second opinion will not involve any pain — and can be done by mail — so there will be no need for traveling.

For some benign tumors, surgery may be curative. For malignant tumors, surgery may relieve symptoms caused by too much pressure in the brain and allow time for other treatments to work. Malignant tumors can grow so fast that without surgery, other treatments might not have the time to work. Surgery is also an opportunity to try a treatment that requires direct access to the brain.

Surgery is performed by a neurosurgeon. However, a general neurosurgeon may not have adequate experience in the removal of brain tumors and may be less informed regarding current treatment therapies. Most neurosurgeons do not see many brain tumors. You need to find one that specializes in brain tumors. Check out the websites of potential neurosurgeons to make sure that "brain tumors" is listed as one of the main areas of expertise.

An "expert" is defined as one who performs a minimum of 25 surgeries per year; typically these neurosurgeons are associated at some level with major brain tumor centers. Studies indicate that major brain tumor centers and/or surgical teams that perform 50 or more surgeries a year exhibit better survival rates and fewer complications.

"Brain surgery" sounds like a very scary thing. It is. But as previously mentioned, it is now much safer and easier than ever. Advances in 3D computer-guided imaging, intraoperative imaging with ultrasound or MRI, brain mapping, and small endoscopes allow surgeons to remove many tumors that used to be considered inoperable. There are still some tumors that are too dangerous to remove because of their size or location, but the limits are shrinking every year. If you are told that your tumor is inoperable, get another opinion.

Debulking (dee-BUL-king): *Surgical removal of as much of a tumor as possible. Debulking may increase the chance that chemotherapy or radiation therapy will kill all the tumor cells. It may also be done to relieve symptoms or help the patient live longer. Also called tumor debulking.*

The virtualtrials.com website hosts a video library, with up-to-date videos from medical and patient brain tumor conferences that cover all aspects of brain tumor treatment, from radiation therapy to the latest chemotherapeutic drugs. To view a menu of these videos and to start watching them, go to: www.virtualtrials.com/video.cfm.

Laser ablation therapy

Laser ablation therapy is a relatively new yet proven minimally invasive technology that uses precise, high-intensity laser energy to destroy tissue in the brain, while limiting injury to healthy tissue. Laser ablation therapy can be used with lesions in many locations in the brain, near the surface or deep inside. During the procedure, physicians use MRI to guide the laser device precisely to the lesion. The procedure has been used with thousands of patients and has been shown to be successful in reducing or removing diseased tissue. The technical name for the procedure is Laser Interstitial Thermal Therapy (LITT).

Unlike traditional brain surgery, LITT does not require a large opening in the head. Instead, physicians make a small hole in the skull, about as big around as a pencil. While the head is secured in place, they guide a small laser device (probe) through that hole precisely into the lesion. The probe delivers laser light energy to heat up and destroy the lesion — a process called ablation. The precise nature of the procedure helps to lessen the likelihood of harm to nearby healthy brain tissue.

LITT might be prescribed when a brain tumor is situated in a place that could be difficult to treat with conventional surgery without harming the brain and the person's ability to function. The LITT tool that is most commonly used is the NeuroBlate system, and information about it can be found at the following website: mybrainsurgeryoptions.com.

Radiation therapy

Radiation therapy is performed under the care of a radiation oncologist or neurosurgeon typically after surgery or in cases where surgery is not an option due to the location or size of the brain tumor. The tumor and a small margin around the tumor are usually targeted by a powerful beam of radiation. The radiation disrupts the DNA of the cells that are reproducing.

Because tumor cells reproduce much more frequently than normal brain cells, they are more affected by radiation than normal cells. Normal cells are also better able to repair damage caused by radiation than tumor cells. Breaking up the course of radiation into a number of smaller treatments called "**fractionation**" instead of one big treatment takes

5

advantage of the differences between tumor cells and normal cells, giving normal cells enough time to repair themselves between treatments. For the standard-of-care treatment, a course of radiation therapy involves a few minutes of treatment five times a week for 6 weeks, together with concomitant administration of Temodar. Side effects of radiation can be mild to severe and include skin burning and peeling, swelling (edema), diarrhea, and nerve damage. There are many types of radiation:

- **Whole brain radiation.** This application of radiation to the entire brain is usually only used when there are multiple tumors, especially metastatic brain tumors. In the past, it was used for all brain tumors, but more focused forms of radiation are now usually administered.

- **Conformal 3D radiation.** This form of radiation therapy targets the tumor and a small margin of tissue outside the tumor with "conventional" external beam radiation. Such targeting spares more of the normal brain from radiation damage and is now standard of care for most brain tumors.

- **Interstitial radiation therapy (also known as brachytherapy).** This form of radiation therapy is delivered directly to the tumor bed by implantation of radioactive material. It may be in the form of radioactive seeds implanted permanently or temporarily. Or it may be by means of the Gliasite Radiation Therapy System, whereby a balloon implanted into the tumor cavity is later filled with a radioactive liquid for a few days and is then later removed. The advantage of such approaches is delivery of a much higher dose of radiation exactly to the site where it is needed. The disadvantage is that surgery is needed to implant these devices. A variation on brachytherapy is targeted administration of a radioactive substance combined with a monoclonal antibody. The antibody seeks out the tumor cells, dragging along the radiation to where it is needed. The use of monoclonal antibodies to deliver radioactive substances is experimental but shows a lot of promise.

- **Stereotactic radiosurgery (SRS).** Although no "knife" or incision is used to expose the brain during SRS but rather a precise high-dose beam of radiation, SRS is considered "surgical" because of the degree of change that takes place after the procedure.

Fractionation (FRAK-shuh-NAY-shun): *Dividing the total dose of radiation therapy into several smaller, equal doses delivered over a period of several days.*

SRS can involve one treatment session or several (fractionated) sessions over a period of several days or weeks, assisted by computer-aided planning. SRS delivers a much higher dose of radiation to the target than conventional radiation therapy. For some low-grade tumors, SRS can be curative. For metastatic tumors, there is a good chance that it can permanently control individual tumors. SRS is also sometimes used as a boost at the end of conventional radiation therapy or for small tumor recurrences. Many different manufacturers have developed devices for administering SRS. Some of the notable brands are Gamma Knife, Novalis System, Linac, and Cyberknife. Each SRS device has its own advantages and disadvantages. **Just know that if you are told your tumor is too large or the wrong shape for SRS, get another opinion from a doctor who uses a different type of SRS device.** For example, the Gamma Knife has a size limit of 3 cm to 4 cm, which other SRS devices do not have.

- **Proton radiation.** This form of radiation therapy uses hydrogen proton particles instead of x-ray or gamma rays. The main advantage is that it delivers energy to a better defined area. That is useful when a tumor is against an important structure, such as the optic nerve, or when a tumor is in a child, for whom you want to limit radiation exposure to as much of the normal brain as possible. Only a few centers in the United States use proton radiation. The cost is significantly higher than standard radiation therapies.

- **Carbon ion.** The use of carbon ion particles is another form of radiation therapy. The advantage of carbon ion particles over proton particles is that they have a higher biological efficiency — that is, they are better at killing cancer cells. However, carbon ion radiation is not as precise as proton radiation in limiting damage behind the target. Carbon ion radiation is used in Germany, Japan, and other countries, but not yet in the United States.

- **Boron neutron capture therapy.** With this form of targeted radiation, a boron compound, which has a higher affinity to tumor tissue than to nontumor tissue, is injected into the patient, and then a neutron beam is directed at the tumor area. The neutron beam reacts with the boron to kill the cells that attracted the boron. There was limited success with this therapy in the past, but with the recent development of better ways to apply boron to the tumor, the therapy is showing promise. It is available in Europe and Asia but considered experimental in the United States.

The virtualtrials.com website of the Musella Foundation has a section that attempts to explain in plain English each of the latest brain tumor treatments in general use, with a brief overview of each, then details on the treatment and where to find it. This section is frequently updated. To access this section, go to: www.virtualtrials.com/noteworth.cfm.

Chemotherapy

Chemotherapy is the use of drugs to kill tumor cells. Chemotherapy drugs work in several ways, each unique to the type of treatment recommended, by (1) destroying the tumor's DNA directly; (2) restricting the tumor cell's ability to divide, grow, and invade healthy tissue; or (3) blocking the blood supply to the tumor itself and inhibiting the growth of new blood vessels that would otherwise feed the tumor.

Chemotherapy is traditionally administered orally as pills or intravenously. New forms of delivery specifically to the brain tumor site show great promise because they bypass the blood-brain barrier, thereby getting a higher concentration of drug to where it is needed and reducing harmful side effects to the body. Of the novel forms of delivery, the three most interesting approaches are the Gliadel wafer, which is implanted during surgery; convection-enhanced delivery; and super-selective intra-arterial infusion. Of these three delivery approaches, only the Gliadel wafer is currently FDA approved and available; the others are still experimental.

Chemotherapy can be administered before, during, and/or after radiation therapy. As noted above, for high grade malignant gliomas, standard-of-care treatment is surgery first with or without implantation of the Gliadel wafer, then radiation therapy and chemotherapy with Temodar at the same time for 6 weeks, followed by 6 months of Temodar with alternating electric field therapy. The common side effects of chemotherapy include nausea, weakness and fatigue, dehydration, and low white blood cell counts, which increase the risk of infection. Because a simple cavity or early gum infection (gingivitis) can quickly escalate into an acute infection for patients undergoing chemotherapy, you should obtain a thorough dental examination prior to beginning chemotherapy and follow up frequently with the dental care team.

At the beginning of this chapter, the importance of genetic testing of your tumor tissue was emphasized. If you are undergoing chemotherapy after surgery, genetic testing is especially important because there are genetic markers in tumors that can indicate potential drug resistance. In particular, an enzyme produced in tumors by what is called the MGMT gene makes chemotherapy with agents like Temodar and BCNU (used in Gliadel wafers) less effective. Because not all patients have active MGMT genes that produce this enzyme, you should find out whether you do.

FDA-approved chemotherapy drugs

As noted above, some FDA-approved chemotherapy drugs have been approved specifically for the treatment of brain tumors, and other FDA-approved chemotherapy drugs have been approved for the treatment of other types of cancer but not specifically for the treatment of brain tumors. When these latter FDA-approved drugs are used for brain tumors, they are used "off-label."

- **Temodar (temozolomide).** Temodar is an oral alkylating chemotherapy. It is the standard-of-care chemotherapeutic agent for the treatment of newly diagnosed brain tumors, and it is approved by the FDA specifically for that use.

- **PCV.** PCV is a combination of the three chemotherapeutic drugs procarbazine, CCNU, and vincristine. Delivered in part orally and in part intravenously, PCV was the most popular treatment for brain tumors before Temodar came along. It is now a second-line treatment for when Temodar does not work, but it is sometimes used as a first-line treatment for oligodendroglioma. A test is available to tell whether an oligo-dendroglioma will be sensitive to PCV.

- **Irinotecan.** Irinotecan is an intravenous chemotherapy agent approved for colon cancer but being tried for brain tumors. There is hope that a high concentration of Irino-tecan at the tumor site may allow it to work better.

- **High-dose tamoxifen.** Tamoxifen is approved for use to prevent the recurrence of breast cancer. When used for brain tumors, it is administered in much higher doses. Only a small percentage of brain tumor patients respond to this agent, but when they do, it can sometimes work miracles. This oral drug has relatively minor side effects, such as a small increased risk of blood clots, but its use does put women into menopause immediately, for it is a type of antiestrogen. Some doctors add tamoxifen to other treatments so no opportunity is lost. Others use tamoxifen as a last resort. There is a report that inducing a hypothyroid state in the patient makes tamoxifen work better. Tamoxifen was used more frequently before so many other choices became available, but it is still worth a look.

- **VP-16.** VP-16 (also called etoposide) is an oral chemotherapy with minimal side effects. It is now used as a second-line treatment for high-grade gliomas.

- **BCNU** and **CCNU.** These two drugs are the oldest treatments for brain tumors, and they have been approved by the FDA for that indication. BCNU (also called carmustine) is given intravenously, and CCNU is usually given orally. They are basically different forms of the same drug. Some doctors use these drugs instead of Temodar or alternate them with Temodar. The major side effect of these drugs is pulmonary fibrosis, so a breathing test is required before starting them and frequently afterwards.

- **Gliadel wafer.** The Gliadel wafer is a biodegradable polymer impregnated with BCNU. The wafers are placed by neurosurgeons up against the walls of the tumor cavity before the membrane, skull, and scalp are closed after the tumor is removed. The wafers slowly dissolve over several days, releasing BCNU. The drug penetrates into the surrounding brain tissue to treat microscopic tumor cells left behind after surgery in order to prevent and delay regrowth of the tumor. Gliadel wafers are the only high-grade glioma treatment that delivers a chemotherapeutic drug directly at the brain tumor site without needing to cross the blood-brain barrier.

Pharmaceutical companies often have sponsored programs to help pay for any medication not covered under your insurance plan, such as a use that would be considered "off label." Ask your treating physician if the pharmaceutical company making the medication has such a plan available. Plans are usually income based, but most physicians will not know the income cut-offs, as only the pharmaceutical company will have that information.

For help paying for medications, two resources are available:
- NeedyMeds, a nonprofit information resource devoted to helping people in need find assistance programs to help them afford their medications and costs related to health care (www.needymeds.org).
- The Musella Foundation co-pay assistance program can help patients pay for one or more of the following treatments: Avastin, Gliadel wafer, Temodar, and the Optune device (www.braintumorcopays.org).

Anti-angiogenesis drugs

Anti-angiogenesis drugs inhibit the growth of new blood vessels to feed the tumor. Avastin is an FDA-approved anti-angiogenesis drug for treatment of recurrent GBM brain tumors. Avastin sometimes has an immediate (within a few days) effect and a remarkable impact on MRI scans and patient well-being — at least for a while. In recent studies, the addition of Avastin to Temodar for patients with newly diagnosed GBM improved progression-free survival but did not improve overall survival. Some doctors think Avastin is best held in reserve for use at the time of recurrence.

Gene therapy / viral therapy

Gene therapy is the insertion of a gene (usually carried by a virus) into a cell in order to replace a defective cell gene or install a new gene that can cause the cell to produce a protein for fighting a tumor. Gene therapy trials for brain tumors have not to date yielded exciting results. However, there is renewed interest in gene therapy because of the Tocagen Toca 5 trial.

- **The Toca 5 trial.** The basic concept of this trial is injection of the Toca 511 virus into a tumor. This virus was designed to infect only brain tumor cells, leaving normal cells alone. When the Toca 511 virus infects a tumor cell, it adds a gene to the cell. This gene, in turn, encodes for an enzyme that can convert an antibiotic drug (Toca FC) into toxic chemotherapy (5-FU) selectively in the tumor. The antibiotic Toca FC drug is then given orally every few weeks, and it kills the tumor cells that have enough copies of the enzyme to convert Toca FC to 5-FU. Tumor cells infected with the Toca 511 virus that do not yet produce enough enzyme serve as a reservoir to continue to spread the infection. With ingestion of the Toca FC antibiotic, the process starts over again and is repeated until the entire tumor is potentially gone. Toca-511 gene therapy is still in clinical trials.

Immunotherapy / vaccine therapy

Immunotherapy, including vaccines, is one of the most exciting areas of research for brain tumors. A large number of different immunotherapy clinical trials for brain tumors are currently underway. Immunotherapy is the treatment of disease by enhancing the body's immune system response to a pathogen. There are two main types of vaccine approaches:

- **Personalized vaccines.** Personalized vaccines require that a tumor specimen be sent to a laboratory to identify tumor-specific antigens (proteins) on the surface of the tumor cells. Specific tumor antigens are combined with patient dendritic cells — a type of immune cell found in tissue — to form a personalized vaccine. These antigens stimulate an immune response, activating killer T immune cells to destroy the tumor. Results from some early vaccine trials have reported that patients with GBM receiving a personalized vaccine survive more than twice as long as patients receiving just standard-of-care treatment. **Please note:** If you are interested in treatment with a personalized vaccine, you must make arrangements before surgery to have the vaccine made or to have frozen tissue stored so that you can have the vaccine made later.

- **"Stock" vaccines.** These vaccines use a different approach. They find the most common targets on the tumors and create a vaccine against them. One trial, called ICT-107, selected six of the most popular tumor targets from which to make one vaccine. Early results of this trial have shown that the vaccine was extremely accurate: 75% of patients had all six targets on their tumors, and 100% had at least three of the six targets on their tumors. To date, the results have been mixed: the early phase 1 trial had remarkable results, but the larger phase 2 trial found a much smaller (although still impressive) improvement in progression-free and overall survival. A large phase 3 trial of ICT-107, which is underway, should tell us how well this vaccine works. Another virus under investigation is PVS-RIPO, a man-made form of the live polio vaccine. Polio viruses can attach to and infect malignant glioma cells. Once inside the glioma cell, the viruses destroy the cells, which causes an immune response so that other tumor cells can be recognized and destroyed by the body's immune system. Recently, the FDA granted PVS-RIPO a breakthrough therapy designation as a potential treatment for patients with recurrent GBM, citing evidence from an ongoing phase 1 study.

Tumor-treating fields

Optune, previously known as NovoTTF-100A system, is a wearable battery-operated device that has recently been approved by the FDA for the treatment of newly diagnosed GBM. The FDA approval is for use in combination with Temodar maintenance therapy after initial concomitant treatment with radiation therapy and Temodar (the standard-of care treatment known as the "Stupp protocol"). Optune has also been approved by the FDA for treatment of recurrent GBM.

The Optune device delivers alternating electric fields (tumor-treating fields) through four insulated transducer arrays. These arrays are worn on a shaved scalp and are connected with a battery-operated field-generating device, which can be carried as a travel case or backpack. The transducer arrays can be worn continuously for 3 to 4 days before they need to be removed for hygienic care of the scalp, re-shaving of hair, and reapplication with a new set of arrays. Loose-knit wigs, hats, or other head coverings can all be worn over the arrays. The figure on the opposite page depicts a man wearing Optune arrays while opening the Optune travel case/backpack.

For a full overview of Optune, with frequent updates, visit the Optune website: www.optune.com. Because Optune is a new treatment, this website can help you find doctors in your area who are certified in its use.

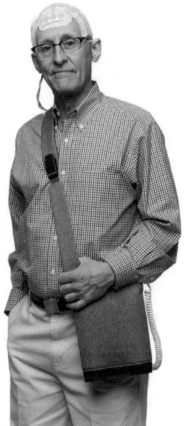

5

The Optune array and carry case / backpack. Courtesy of Novocure, Inc. © Novocure 2016. All rights reserved.

An addition to the standard of care
The phase 3 randomized clinical trial of Optune in combination with standard-of-care Temodar therapy for treatment of patients with newly diagnosed GBM was hailed by its lead investigator, Roger Stupp, MD, as having "spectacular results" and as promising a "new standard of care for patients suffering from glioblastoma." The scientific report of the phase III randomized Optune trial in patients with newly diagnosed GBM, entitled "Maintenance therapy with tumor-treating fields plus temozolomide vs temozolomide alone for glioblastoma: a randomized clinical trial," was published in the prestigious *Journal of the American Medical Association*. To see the published report, go to: jama.jamanetwork.com/article.aspx?articleid=2475463.

Tumor-treating fields selectively disrupt the division of cells by delivering low-intensity, intermediate-frequency alternating electric fields. These alternating electric fields affect only dividing cells; non-dividing cells are spared. Since tumor-treating fields do not enter the bloodstream like drugs, they do not affect cells in other parts of the body. The most common side effects seen with Optune are mild-to-moderate scalp irritation from wearing the device and possibly headache.

A large phase 3 randomized controlled trial has been conducted to compare the use of Optune plus Temodar versus the use of Temodar alone for patients with newly diagnosed GBM who had received radiation therapy with concurrent Temodar. The FDA actually stopped this phase 3 trial early because there were clearly evident increases in progression-free and overall survival in the Optune plus Temodar group compared with the Temodar-only group. The FDA stated that all of the patients in the trial should be allowed to benefit from Optune treatment. This FDA action might be the first time ever that a brain tumor trial was stopped early because a treatment was found to be so clearly effective.

The virtualtrials.com website of the Musella Foundation has separate sections, each with extensive information, about several of the key brain tumor treatments. Be sure to visit each of the following sections for the latest updates about these treatments:
- Brain tumor vaccines (www.virtualtrials.com/vaccines.cfm)
- Gliadel wafer (www.virtualtrials.com/gliadel)
- Optune (www.virtualtrials.com/novocure)
- Temodar (www.virtualtrials.com/temodar)
- Toca 511 & Toca FC (www.virtualtrials.com/tocagen)

Long-term side effects

In the past, the consequences of long-term side effects were never a big concern because people did not live long enough for them to be a concern. Luckily, there has been a steady rise in the number of long-term survivors of brain tumors. Now long-term side effects have to be considered when choosing a treatment.

Radiation therapy can cause vascular injury and increase the risk of stroke. Unfortunately, stroke is fairly common among long-term survivors of brain tumors and can be either completely asymptomatic or completely devastating, depending on the location. Stroke risk can be reduced by managing risk factors. Please talk to your doctor about stroke risk.

Another long-term side effect of radiation therapy is cognitive loss, which varies with the dose of radiation and the volume and location radiated. Cognitive loss is nearly universal with whole brain radiation. These side effects can be minimized by limiting the treatment to only the site of the tumor and a small margin around the tumor.

Chemotherapy is often associated with long-term infertility, but you can offset this side effect by freezing sperm or eggs before chemotherapy begins. Fertility may be the last thing you are worried about now, but what happens if you want kids a few years from now and cannot have them? Think about it.

Drugs such as BCNU and CCNU can cause pulmonary fibrosis. You have to monitor lung function with these drugs. There are also rare cases of myelodysplasia or "pre-leukemia" conditions related to chemotherapy, particularly in association with alkylating agents like Temodar. So although it remains unclear what the best length of treatment with Temodar is, staying on Temodar forever might not be best either. More research is needed on this question.

Avastin can cause severe high blood pressure, problems with wound healing, and rupture of the intestines. **Report gastrointestinal pain or rectal bleeding to your doctors immediately.** You will need to see your internist regularly to check the rest of your body. Watch for swelling of the legs and feet, pain in the back of the leg, pressure in the chest, or difficulty breathing. Any of these symptoms may indicate a blood clot, and you need to see a doctor immediately. If your doctor is not available, go to an emergency room.

The Brain Tumor Virtual Trial

The Brain Tumor Virtual Trial is a registry managed and run by the Musella Foundation. The virtual trial consists of a database of brain tumor patients, the treatments they are using, and their outcomes. Participants record the treatments that they and their medical teams decide to pursue. We do not tell you what treatments to receive; we just record the outcomes. There is no cost to participate in the virtual trial. The patient or caregiver records information in simple forms on the virtualtrials.com website and posts an update each month. We send email reminders on the first of each month. You also send in a copy of each of your MRI reports (not the MRI films) and pathology reports so that information can be verified. Participants get to view the ongoing results of the project.

The concept behind the Brain Tumor Virtual Trial is to identify which treatments, or which combination of treatments, are working the best. In addition to providing greater insight to researchers about beneficial therapies in the real world, participants also learn how to become expert managers of their own condition. For example, participants can generate reports on the information they entered, such as a graph of their status over time.

For more information on the Brain Tumor Virtual Trial, go to: www.virtualtrials.com/brain/index.cfm. ●

Survivor story #5: Ben Williams

At the age of 50, I had surgery for glioblastoma multiforme (GBM) on March 31, 1995, after an MRI scan in the emergency room the preceding day. The tumor was located in my right parietal cortex and was very large (it was approximately 180 cc and described as the "size of a large orange"). My neurosurgeon later told me that I would have been dead within two weeks had I not had the surgery when I did.

During the first two months after my diagnosis, I spent many hours on the Internet and in our medical school library, learning all that I could about possible treatment options. While I initially entertained boron neutron capture therapy, gene therapy, and radiation-loaded monoclonal antibodies as much more promising than conventional treatment, I finally rejected all of these based on likely problems of various sorts. I therefore opted for conventional chemotherapy but in combination with other agents that seemed likely to improve the effectiveness of chemotherapy over that which typically occurs.

All of my MRI scans since chemotherapy have been free of any sign of tumor. Throughout my first year of treatment I added various nutritional supplements that can be obtained at most health food stores.

The inspiration for the various treatments and health food commodities I have opted for has come from many different sources. Much of it came from my own research on Medline, sometimes after hearing about a treatment in passing from participants in an online support group. I also found the webpage of the Musella foundation as a source of leads to follow up.

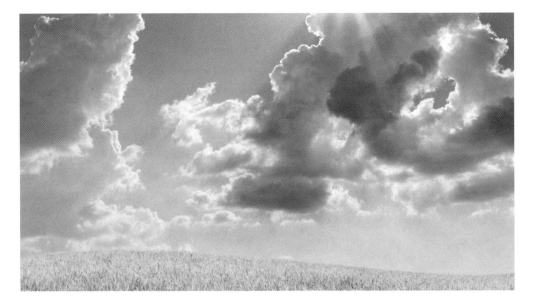

My treatment philosophy has been very similar to the treatment approach that has developed for AIDS. Both HIV and cancer involve biological entities that mutate at high rates, so unless a treatment is almost instantaneously effective, the dynamics of evolution will create new forms that are resistant to whatever the treatment may be. However, if several different treatments are used simultaneously (instead of sequentially, which is typically the case), any given mutation has a much smaller chance of being successful.

A second feature of my treatment philosophy is that any successful treatment will need to be systemic in nature, since it is impossible to identify all of the extensions of the tumor into normal tissue.

Ben Williams, a 21-year survivor of GBM, is the author of the 2002 book *Surviving Terminal Cancer: Clinical Trials, Drug Cocktails, and Other Treatments Your Oncologist Won't Tell You About*. At the virtualtrials.com website, he has posted various updates of this book, including 2014 updates of "Treatment options for malignant gliomas" and "The role of supplements (including anti-oxidants) in cancer treatment." To access these important updates, go to: www.virtualtrials.com/williams.cfm.

5

KEY POINTS

☑ Find an expert neurosurgeon who specializes in brain tumors.

☑ Before surgery begins, ask about genetic tests, drug-resistance tests, enrollment in clinical trials, personalized gene therapy, and the implantation of Gliadel wafers.

☑ The current standard-of-care treatment for newly diagnosed high-grade malignant glioma consists of a combination of up to 5 different treatments, depending on patient and tumor characteristics: (1) surgery; (2) implantation of Gliadel wafers in the tumor cavity during surgery; (3) radiation therapy; (4) oral chemotherapy during and after radiotherapy; and (5) alternating electric field therapy (the Optune device) after radiotherapy. If this standard-of-care treatment is not offered to you, ask why not.

☑ Consider entering a clinical trial.

☑ Enroll in the Brain Tumor Virtual Trial registry managed and run by the Musella Foundation, a database of brain tumor patients, the treatments they are using, and their outcomes.

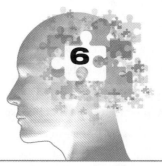

Chapter 6
Alternative and complementary treatments

Discussing alternative and complementary treatments is a little like discussing religion and politics. These topics are hard and emotional, there is often a lot of fear associated with them, and there can be many points of view.

This guide will give you an understanding of alternative and complementary treatments, but as with anything else, the final decision to use them must be yours.

Alternative treatments are treatments that have not yet been proven to work based on scientific testing and are used INSTEAD of mainstream treatments.

Complementary treatments have also not yet been proven to work but are used IN ADDITION to mainstream treatments. Once a treatment has been shown to work, it crosses over from "alternative"/"complementary" to "mainstream."

The mainstream path of treatment development

When someone invents or discovers a treatment that he or she thinks may help with a brain tumor, the path to the treatment's becoming part of mainstream medicine begins with laboratory testing on cell cultures and/or on animals. If the treatment still seems promosing, human trials are started. We discuss clinical trials in another section, but basically the treatment is tested on people with a brain tumor and is compared with either historical controls or with a control group.

The early stages of a trial, when only a few people are tested, cannot really show how well the treatment actually works. All phase III trials have had successful phase I and phase II trials leading up to them. However, most phase III brain tumor trials have failed to show significant benefit compared to standard treatment even though a new tested treatment looked very good in early trials. The reason for this is that the course of a brain tumor is variable. A small percentage of patients will do well no matter what treatment you give them, and the natural history is a roller coaster — you have wild ups and downs. If you happen by chance to select a handful of brain tumor patients who happen to have the right subtype, genetics, age, resection extent, **Karnofsky Performance Status,** and other prognostic factors, and are on the right track of the roller coaster at the time, they may do well in a small trial even if the treatment is not as good as the standard treatment.

The next step is to test the treatment in a large group. This is when you conduct a **randomized clinical trial,** in which patients are assigned by chance to receive treatment with either the new therapy or placebo (an inactive substance that looks just like the new therapy) or standard treatment. Then, when the two groups are compared, you get a much better feel for how the new therapy works, since all the other variables are controlled. The trials need to be repeated a few times on large numbers of patients treated before you will know if the effect is treatment related or chance related.

Statistics are used to try to make sense of the trial results. A number is calculated called the significance level. The number usually chosen as the benchmark is 0.05, which means that there is a 95% chance that the effect seen in the trial was caused by the treatment and not by chance alone. Conversely, this means that if you run 100 trials of a worthless drug, about 5 of those trials may report success even though there is none. This is why multiple trials are needed, and it is best if they are conducted by different centers.

The FDA will approve a drug that is better than standard treatment, or is at least as good as standard treatment, if it has fewer side effects. Once a treatment is approved by the FDA, everyone can get access to it, not just those in clinical trials.

Karnofsky Performance Status (kar-NOF-skee per-FOR-munts STA-tus): *A standard way of measuring the ability of cancer patients to perform ordinary tasks. The Karnofsky Performance scores range from 0 to 100. A higher score means the patient is better able to carry out daily activities. KPS may be used to determine a patient's prognosis, to measure changes in a patient's ability to function, or to decide if a patient could be included in a clinical trial.*

Randomized clinical trial (RAN-duh-mized KLIH-nih-kul TRY-ul): *A study in which the participants are assigned by chance to separate groups that compare different treatments; neither the researchers nor the participants can choose which group. Using chance to assign people to groups means that the groups will be similar and that the treatments they receive can be compared objectively. At the time of the trial, it is not known which treatment is best. It is the patient's choice to be in a randomized trial.*

How alternative treatments are developed

An alternative treatment is developed when someone has an idea that a certain treatment may help a brain tumor, or the researchers notice that a brain tumor survivor has tried a certain treatment. They then try the treatment on a few more brain tumor patients and see that some of them get better. (As mentioned before, some brain tumor patients are on the upswing of the roller coaster and would have been doing better even without the treatment.)

At that point, the researchers are convinced the treatment works, and they try to promote it so that more people can benefit from it. In many cases, these are the most well-meaning people with the best of motives. They saw something work in a few patients and want others to do well also. However, the difference is in the science. At this point, it would be good to follow the mainstream path and do rigorous trials of a new treatment, and if it passes the tests, the novel treatment would become mainstream and help everyone. However, that is often not the path taken. Instead, many promoters of alternative and complementary therapies skip the proof and go on to marketing. They use individual case reports or small trials to justify the treatment.

On the Internet, we read about many of these types of treatments, which introduces a huge new problem: selection bias. This means that you hear from and see the people who do well with a treatment but you do not see the ones who died. For example, if the standard treatment for a brain tumor has an average survival period of 18 months (and some of the experimental treatments more than double that), an alternative treatment needs to reach that point to just say it is as good as standard treatment.

Put another way: If you take 1000 patients and put them on standard treatment, you would expect 500 of them to be alive in 18 months. If you take the same 1000 patients and give them a treatment that is half as effective as standard treatment, you would expect to see 250 alive at 18 months. If you see 250 people telling you that this miracle alternative treatment worked for them, you may tend to believe them. But you are not seeing the 750 who died — they can't tell you that it didn't work for them. So, at that point, what question should you ask? If they tell you they have 250 18-month brain tumor survivors, ask out of how many that started? If it is 250 out of 250, it is a miracle. If it is 250 out of 1000, it is only half as good as standard treatment.

Frequently, those who recommend alternative treatments for serious illness will say "It doesn't hurt to try since the standard treatment does not result in a cure." This statement is erroneous, since even if the treatment itself is not toxic or dangerous, the use of such treatment often works against the science-based treatment, or sometimes is even used as a sole approach (stopping the scientific treatment that, while not curative, may temporarily bring some relief to patients).

Also, the high cost of alternative treatment, usually not covered by health insurance, can cause serious financial pain to families and patients who desperately cling to straws of a "cure" offered by those who sell these nonscientific treatments.

There are "red lights" to watch out for when dealing with non-scientifically based treatments. The following are some of the most common "red lights" associated with alternative treatments:

- They are proprietary (available from one source or a limited number of sources) and are not available on the standard pharmaceutical market (which is subject to government supervision and regulation).

- They are expensive, and patients and their families must usually "pay up" in advance before the treatment can be started or continued. Most true clinical trials are licensed and supervised by government entities and are backed with public or private grants so that patients pay little or nothing for the treatment. Most legitimate studies are run in or by major universities or other institutions of higher learning, whereas the majority of alternative schemes are run by for-profit entities.

- The results of the alternative programs have not stood the test of review by a **peer-reviewed scientific journal** (in most cases, the data have not even been submitted to peer-reviewed scientific journals for publication). The alternative programs rely on "testimonials" by patients or former patients, and these are highly unreliable, especially when the diagnosis (of cancer) has not been based on scientific diagnostic techniques, such as pathological examination of tissue.

- There is often a tendency for the providers of alternative treatment to speak ill of traditional scientific medicine, frequently asserting that organized medicine is involved in a conspiracy to force patients to get orthodox treatment for the economic gain of the medical profession.

Peer-reviewed scientific journal (peer-ree-VYOOD SY-en-TIH-fik JER-nul):
A publication that contains original articles that have been written by scientists and evaluated for technical and scientific quality and correctness by other experts in the same field.

Brain tumor patients contact us frequently at the Musella Foundation. Many of them have tried just about every alternative treatment ever proposed for brain tumors. Some of them do well. Most do not. We track them with our Brain Tumor Virtual Trial project. **Analyzing our data for this project, we found that not one of the alternative treatments reported had any effect on the outcome of the cases**.

We still keep an eye on the patients who do not join the project. The ones that use mainstream treatments do better than the ones who use alternative treatments alone. We have seen many people decline and die rapidly when refusing standard treatments. They usually change their minds near the end and start standard treatments, but of course it is too late. Unfortunately, they then blame the standard treatments for the death.

However, when it comes to complementary treatments, when you use mainstream treatments but add to them, you may see some positive results. There may be some complementary treatments that do help with treatment side effects and possibly may make treatments more effective. However, keep in mind that if you feel a complementary treatment is powerful enough to change the course of your tumor in a positive way, it is just as likely — or more so — to be able to change it in a negative way. The body is very complicated. You cannot predict what would happen if you change one thing, because one small change can upset the delicate balance of the body and have unseen consequences. The only way to tell is by trying it in a well-designed trial. Proponents may say there is no money in it so no one would fund the trial. That is not true. The Musella Foundation, as well as most of the over 100 other brain tumor foundations, fund research projects like this.

Conspiracy theories may be put to rest by these two simple thoughts: (1) there is no way the medical industry is organized enough to keep away from the public a cure that would be the biggest money maker in the world; and (2) there are many researchers who dedicate their lives to finding the cure.

Patients need to learn to ask the right critical questions:

- WHAT exactly is this treatment?
- WHO has received it?
- HOW MANY brain tumor patients have had documented responses, and how many patients have tried it?
- HOW are responses assessed?
- WHY is it not given as part of mainstream practice in the United States?

- HOW was the diagnosis of brain tumor made? In some countries, MRI scans are not routine for brain tumor patients, and even if there is an MRI, there are many diseases that look similar to a brain tumor. A biopsy is the best way to tell if the diagnosis is a brain tumor and which type it is.
- HAVE the treatment results been published in a peer-reviewed journal? If not, why not? ●

KEY POINTS

☑ Alternative treatments have not yet been proved to work based on scientific testing and are used **instead of** mainstream treatments.

☑ Complementary treatments have not yet been proved to work based on scientific testing, but they are used **in addition to** mainstream treatments.

☑ There are several "red lights" to watch out for when dealing with non-scientifically based treatments – few sources for the products; an expensive cost; reliance on patient "testimonials" rather than publication of data in peer-reviewed scientific journals; and conspiracy talk.

☑ Learn to ask the right critical questions about alternative and complementary treatments. What is it? Who and how many have received it? How were responses assessed? Why is it not part of US mainstream practice? How was the diagnosis of brain tumor confirmed? And have the treatment data been published in a peer-reviewed scientific journal?

6

Survivor story #6

On November 29, 2006, after she had suffered from headaches for more than a week, I took my wife to the hospital. Something was terribly wrong. After the initial examination, including CT and MRI scans, it was revealed that a potentially bleeding mass was present in her brain, and there was significant swelling and a midline shift between the two halves of her brain. After much prayer and consideration, we opted to have surgery performed right where we were instead of traveling to another hospital.

On December 1, 2006, the excellent neurosurgeon removed all of the "visible" tumor. To our amazement, my wife was eating ice cream 3 hours after surgery. The tumor was glioblastoma multiforme (GBM). The pathology was confirmed after the tumor was sent to Duke University Medical Center for a second opinion. My wife underwent 30 radiation treatments with concurrent low-dose Temodar chemotherapy beginning December 26, 2006.

My wife has thrived since surgery and is currently on a 5-day-on, 23-day-off monthly Temodar cycle. Every two months we travel to the National Cancer Institute to see a neuro-oncologist who evaluates her MRI scans and makes suggestions. Between this physician and our local oncologist, we have received excellent medical care.

My wife has now passed 28 months since the diagnosis and removal of her GBM. She has resumed a full schedule of activity and even works out occasionally. The prayers of many faithful people have sustained us and helped. There is hope, even in the face of a GBM diagnosis.

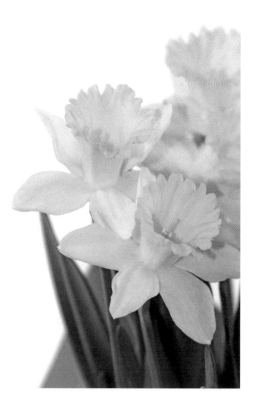

Update in February 2013. My wife has just completed 12 more rounds of Temodar, she is now 14 months out since a recurrence of her brain tumor, but she has survived for over 6 years since her first GBM. She continues to work full time and is doing well considering all that she has been through.

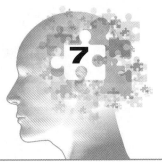

Chapter 7
Common medicines
for treating symptoms

In the treatment of brain tumors, not unlike the treatment of any other acute or chronic illness, a variety of medications are used to combat symptoms, such as pain, fatigue, swelling, and seizures. The medications may include antibiotics, steroids, analgesics or narcotics, and anticonvulsants. It is necessary to take responsibility for your medications to ensure your safety.

As your medical team will be made up of physicians from various specialties, all of whom may prescribe different medications or alter dosages in the context of your care, it is vital that you keep ongoing and accurate (up-to-date) records in your treatment binder regarding your medications, including:

- Medications you're currently taking (including dosages) and who is responsible for monitoring you (prescribing physician) or providing refills. This information can be very helpful to a caregiver seeking information or assistance on your behalf.
- Medications you have taken in the past, noting their value (e.g., "was most helpful for sleep").
- Medications discontinued due to negative side effects.
- Any allergic or adverse reactions, mild or otherwise, noted in RED.

You should always:

- Ask your doctors to review your list of current medications prior to prescribing something new.
- Check to ensure that the recommended drug is covered on your insurance plan's drug formulary, or if you'll need a prior authorization.
- To avoid receiving the wrong medication at the pharmacy (a growing concern), write down the specific medication and dosage as stated on your prescription before

submitting it to a pharmacist and compare this information to the label on the bottle you receive to ensure it is the same drug as stated on the prescription.

• Your prescription might be filled with a **generic** substitution if your doctor did not prescribe it to be "dispensed as written." If the medication you receive is different from what was written on the original prescription by your physician, ask the pharmacist. Also ask the pharmacist for his/her thoughts on the generic. Most generic drugs are okay to use, but for some drugs that have a very narrow effectiveness range, it may be worthwhile to pay the extra for the brand name or insist on the same brand of generic each time.

Whenever possible, having all your prescriptions filled through a single pharmacy source can be a safeguard against medical errors, preventing adverse drug interactions, as most pharmacies now use computer systems that automatically flag dangerous interactions based upon your previous medications. Should your physician fail to recall a particular medication that might present a problem, chances are your pharmacist will catch it. Still, asking your physician(s) to review your medication sheet in your treatment binder — each and every time a new drug is prescribed — is an important, life-saving step.

It is important that you understand the side effects and drug interactions of all the medications you are prescribed. Most of the drugs we use have very scary package inserts and list every side effect ever reported to happen in people who were taking the drugs — whether the drug caused it or not. Our point is to be aware of the most common side effects and watch for them, not to be scared away from using the drugs. Additional information regarding your medications and drug interactions can be found at websites like Drugs.com (www.drugs.com).

The following is a general list of medications commonly used to treat symptoms and/or conditions caused by a brain tumor itself, or resulting from surgery and/or other standardized treatments of brain tumors. Many of the significant/common side effects associated with a particular medication are noted, but the list may be incomplete. Your physician may recommend medications not covered within this general guide. You are advised to thoroughly discuss and understand all the benefits and side effects with your physician before a prescription is issued. Physicians are often creatures of habit — ask about alternative medications and why your physician would choose the recommended medication over another. This is a general overview. Always ask your doctor before taking anything, even over the counter pain medications.

Generic (jeh-NAYR-ik): *Official nonbrand names by which medicines are known. Generic names usually refer to the chemical name of the drug.*

Medications for pain relief

Because the brain itself does not feel pain, studies show that physicians treating patients for brain tumors often overlook pain. However, pain as a by-product of disease or due to complications from surgery or other forms of treatment is very real and deserves real attention. Headaches from brain inflammation or tension, scalp sutures, muscular pain and hairline fractures due to steroid therapy, and pressure points on arms and hips from extended bed rest require medication. Pain left untreated can slow healing, deplete emotional reserves, exacerbate depression and sleep deprivation, and detract from your quality of life.

Mild pain. The lowest level of pain can usually be managed with Tylenol, Advil, or Aleve. (Note that aspirin can affect how fast your blood clots, which may be bad if you need surgery, or good as it prevents blood clots. Always ask your doctor about it first.)

Moderate pain. More powerful prescription medication, such as Percocet (the combination of oxycodone and acetaminophen) and Percodan (the combination of oxycodone and aspirin), can be taken as directed by a physician.

Severe pain. Codeine, Vicodin (the combination of hydrocodone and acetaminophen), oxycodone, and stronger, morphine-type medications are typically long acting and are taken less frequently. Many also come in "patch" form for slow absorption and continuous relief. Ritalin (methylphenidate) is used to treat attention-deficit hyperactivity disorder. If taken in small doses with pain medication, Ritalin can increase the narcotic effect (enhancing pain relief) while reducing the drowsiness commonly associated with these drugs. Ritalin has also been shown to benefit patients who suffer from fatigue. According to package inserts for drugs that contain morphine, such drugs should not be used in patients with brain tumors. However, they are still commonly used, and the benefits may outweigh the risks when you are in severe pain. Discuss any concerns you might have with your physician.

7

Medications for swelling

Steroids are powerful anti-inflammatory drugs typically prescribed to reduce swelling in the brain (cerebral **edema**) before and/or after surgery, during radiation treatments, or to relieve symptoms such as memory loss and limb (arm/leg) weakness caused by brain swelling. While common, swelling can be harmful if excessive and must be controlled.

Synthetic steroids such as Decadron and Hexadrol (dexamethasone) are man-made hormones similar to cortisol, which is produced naturally by your body. Taken orally, these

---

Edema (eh-DEE-muh): *Swelling caused by excess fluid in body tissues.*

To get additional information about any medication, go to the drug information site of the National Institutes of Health, Medline Plus: www.nlm.nih.gov/medlineplus/druginformation.html.

steroids create higher levels in the body than what is normally secreted, reducing inflammation but also causing the body to temporarily stop natural production on its own. For this reason, it is very important to "wean" yourself (cut back slowly) when stopping oral steroid therapy. Always follow your physician's recommended schedule for reducing dosages. During this reduction period, your body will slowly come back "on line" and begin to produce normal cortisol levels again. You should never abruptly stop taking steroid medication, because in extreme cases, going cold turkey can cause sudden death, as the body is not yet ready to resume full production of cortisol on its own, a necessary and vital hormone.

While the benefits of steroids are undeniable, often unmatched by any other medication, they are not without short and long-term side effects.

Long-term side effects can include (but are not limited to) diabetes, muscle pain/weakness, osteoporosis (bone loss) leading to fractures, and susceptibility to infections. Short-term effects can include (but are not limited to) increased appetite, weight gain, and indigestion; swollen or "moon-faced" appearance; stretch marks, rash/flushing of skin, and acne; increase in blood sugar; brittle bones; depression and/or behavioral changes; anxiety and/or paranoia; and suppressed immune system.

Other oral steroidal therapies include prednisone or prednisolone. While not as strong as Decadron or Hexadrol, side effects are generally the same, although perhaps not as severe in most cases. Diamox (acetazolamide) is another type of medication that can sometimes be used to reduce swelling without the side effects of steroids.

Medications for reducing seizures

Roughly 30 to 40 percent of patients will experience some level of seizure activity and require medication to reduce electrical responses in the brain. Due to the location and/or size of some tumors, many neurosurgeons will prescribe anti-seizure medication as a matter of routine before, during, and/or after surgery when the risk of seizure is considered high. In the past, all brain tumor patients were put on anti-seizure medications routinely for life, but since they can have a lot of side effects, *many doctors now try to do without these drugs until seizures occur.*

In some cases, a seizure will appear as something slight and quick — muscle or eye twitching, or a sense of being "out of the moment" mentally and/or physically for a brief time, or a blank stare or sudden pause without response. These are called focal seizures. For others, seizures will involve full body activity, often categorized as grand mal seizures.

Most anticonvulsants share common side effects, such as fatigue and dizziness, so for obvious reasons you may be restricted from driving a car or operating dangerous equipment while taking anti-seizure medications, even when seizures have not been documented or have subsided. Other medications and certain foods can prevent proper absorption, so frequent blood draws for proper dosage and serum levels are necessary.

Phenytoin, often prescribed under the brand name Dilantin, is a commonly used medication to prevent full-body seizures in high-risk patients. People metabolize Dilantin differently, so periodic blood levels are taken to ensure that dosages are adequate and stable. Side effects of Dilantin include muscle fatigue, dizziness, and loss of coordination, as well as tooth decay and gum problems. Regular dental checkups and extra attention to oral hygiene are advised. Long-term use of Dilantin can cause a decrease in certain nutrients, such as folic acid and calcium. Ask your physician about supplements if necessary. Dilantin can also interact with other medications, including over-the-counter drugs, birth control pills, and herbal supplements. Dilantin can also make some chemotherapy drugs less effective.

Neurontin (gabapentin) has similar side effects as Dilantin, as well as the side effects of double vision, tremors, and involuntary eye movements. While Neurontin has fewer drug interactions than Dilantin, it does interact with certain antacids, such as Maalox.

Tegretol (carbamazepine) is an anticonvulsant that is also prescribed in the treatment of manic depression and other psychiatric disorders. Effective in its ability to control grand mal seizures, Tegretol must be monitored closely with frequent blood levels, since in rare cases, it may suppress bone marrow production. You should report any onset of a rash to your physician immediately. Tegretol also reduces or increases the effects of many medications. Double vision, pounding or slow heart rate, and nausea are noted side effects with this drug.

Depakote and Depakene (valporic acid or valproate) are commonly prescribed for focal seizures and require periodic blood levels to ensure adequate dosage and guard against liver damage. Because Depakote interacts with many medications, make sure your physician reviews your current medication list, including over-the-counter and herbal supplements, at the time of recommendation.

Phenobarbitol (a barbiturate and strong depressant) and primidone are less frequently prescribed, as the effectiveness of other anticonvulsants can be more easily achieved without the potentially addictive qualities of these drugs.

Keppra (levetiracetam) is a newer anticonvulsant drug. Sometimes it is used alone, and sometimes for difficult cases it is combined with other drugs. Keppra does not interfere with chemotherapy drugs.

Medications for reducing nausea

Nausea is common with brain tumors, as both a part of the disease process itself and as a by-product of radiation and chemotherapy treatment. Zofran (ondansetron) is used to control nausea caused by chemotherapy or radiation. It is usually administered intravenously prior to treatment and can be taken orally after treatment, if necessary. Effective for only a few hours, Zofran is limited to nausea caused by chemotherapy and radiation only and is not to be taken for motion sickness or other generalized conditions related to nausea. While mild in nature, side effects of Zofran include headache, fatigue, diarrhea, and constipation, and the drug may exacerbate pre-existing liver disease.

Kytril (granisetron) is similar to Zofran in both treatment administration and side effects, although it may also cause abdominal pain. It lasts up to 12 hours.

Compazine (prochlorperazine) is a commonly prescribed medication for the treatment of generalized nausea and is given orally, intravenously, or as a suppository. Compazine belongs to a family of antipsychotic agents called "phenothiazines" and may cause drowsiness, low blood pressure, dizziness, constipation, dry mouth, blurred vision, and sensitivity to light. While effective in the management of nausea, Compazine should not be used in conjunction with alcohol, may interact with other medications, and could potentially cause an irreversible condition called tardive dyskinesia — involuntary movements or twitches of the face, tongue, or arm muscles.

Anzemet (dolasetron) is a new anti-nausea drug currently being used with success. Anzemet is given prior to chemotherapy. In some patients, a combination of Anzamet and Decadron prior to chemotherapy works in cases when the older drugs do not provide enough relief.

Haldol (haloperidol) is another antipsychotic medication used to control nausea with risks and side effects similar to those of Compazine. Haldol and Compazine should not be taken without a detailed discussion with your physician. Transderm Scop contains the seasickness drug scopamine, which can sometimes be used for nausea. Transderm Scop is a patch formulation of the drug that is applied to the skin and works for 3 days per patch. A main side effect is dry mouth, which can be a benefit when there is difficulty swallowing and too much saliva is being produced.

There are also many alternative treatments. Some patients report that acupuncture, biofeedback, and hypnosis provide nausea relief with no side effects and are much cheaper than most commonly used drugs.

Medications for improving mood

Being diagnosed with a brain tumor alone is enough to create overwhelming anxiety and stress. It is important to understand that during the course of treatment, intense and seemingly "over-emotional" reactions — such as acute depression, sexual dysfunction, sudden outbursts, and visual or audio hallucination — may be the result of medication or a condition stemming from the tumor itself, not necessarily an emotional response. It is also important to communicate about these emotional changes with your medical team in order to seek proper assistance and guidance to help you distinguish the many moods of treatment and recovery, and to help you cope.

A psychiatrist is a medical doctor who can assist with the mood-related conditions directly caused by the tumor or its treatment. Psychologists can also provide help with coping difficulties and with mild depression due to issues of long-term care, financial strain, or the stress placed upon family and other important relationships. Ask your medical team to refer you to a psychiatrist or psychologist experienced in treating brain tumor patients.

Common antidepressants include Zoloft (sertraline), Paxil (paroxetine), and Prozac (fluoxetine), all of which are from a class of drugs called selective serotonin reuptake inhibitors (SSRIs). Side effects may include sleepiness, tremors, diarrhea, nausea, insomnia, increased sweating, weight loss, and decreased sexual ability. Side effects may be reduced when SSRIs are taken with meals; Zoloft, in particular, should always be taken with food. In some rare cases, anxiety and depression may worsen while taking SSRIs and should be reported to your medical team immediately. Don't let the risk of side effects stop you from trying these drugs. People report a remarkable increase in quality of life when these drugs work.

Herbal remedies may be of some benefit. However, herbal mixtures can adversely interact with other prescription medications and should always be discussed with your medical team for safety and adequate dosing information. If you are thinking of taking hypericin, one of the principal active compounds of St. John's wort, make sure to ask your medical team first, for hypericin can interfere with other drugs.

7

Medications for reducing the formation of blood clots

Brain tumor patients are at a higher than normal risk for developing dangerous blood clots. Blood clots commonly start in the legs as deep vein thrombosis (DVT). Symptoms of DVT may include pain, tenderness, swelling, discoloration of the affected leg, and skin that is warm to the touch. If you develop these symptoms, you must call your doctor and get it checked quickly. Left untreated, blood clots can break away and travel to the lungs where they may cause a pulmonary embolism, which can be rapidly fatal. Symptoms of a pulmonary embolism include sudden shortness of breath, chest pain (worse with breathing), and rapid heart and respiratory rates. If you develop any of these symptoms, you must go to the emergency room immediately.

Medications called anticoagulants help to thin the blood and reduce clotting, the body's normal response to help stop bleeding. Heparin is an anticoagulant that is given by injection, usually for a short period of time to prevent or treat blood clots. Warfarin (commonly referred to as coumadin) is an oral medication that can be taken over a long period of time to prevent blood clots. Aspirin is a milder blood thinner, which some doctors recommend to prevent blood clots.

When you are taking anticoagulants, normal cuts and scrapes may take longer to stop bleeding or heal, and there is an increased risk of the tumor bleeding into the brain — so these drugs are double-edged swords and should be taken exactly as prescribed. Warfarin interacts with many medications and should be discussed thoroughly with your medical team before treatment. Your doctor will also order periodic blood tests to ensure that appropriate medication levels are maintained. Plavix is another commonly used drug that prevents clotting.

It is important to note that changes to your diet can have a negative effect on the blood-thinning measures of anticoagulant medication. Suddenly increasing foods such as spinach in your diet can adversely affect bleeding times. The sudden introduction of fish-oil capsules (which are full of omega-3 fatty acids) as a dietary supplement can also alter bleeding times. While there is no need to eliminate spinach and other healthy items (including supplements) from your daily routine, you are advised to maintain your normal diet and not increase or decrease items significantly or add new supplements without discussing them with your physician. This is not the time to begin a new diet for weight loss without consulting your physician.

It is always a good idea to wear a medical alert bracelet informing medical personnel that you are taking anticoagulants in the case of an emergency. They are widely available in most retail pharmacies and on the Internet, inexpensive, and an important safeguard for your health. ●

KEY POINTS

☑ Because your medical team will be made up of doctors of different specialties, it is vital that you take responsibility for keeping an ongoing and accurate record of the medications you are taking, including their dosage and the names of the physicians who prescribed them.

☑ Always ask your medical team to review your complete list of medications before they prescribe anything new.

☑ If possible, always fill your prescriptions at the same pharmacy to safeguard against medical errors and adverse drug interactions.

☑ Make yourself knowledgeable about the most common possible side effects and drug interactions of the medications you are taking.

7

Survivor story #7

My story begins in September 2008 with dizzy spells and a heightened sensitivity to bright lights. Something just didn't feel right. When I visited my family doctor, he ordered blood work and thought it might be my heart. I was 43 years old and in good health.

Fast forward to October 2 of that year. I woke up at my usual time and got the kids up, feeling fine. At about 8:00 AM I felt dizzy again and began banging into door frames and tripping. I thought I was having a stroke.

I called my husband at work and told him I needed to go to the emergency room. He rushed home and took me. I was sent for a CT scan, and not long after the doctor and nurse came with the news. "You have a 3-cm tumor in your brain."

We were told to go immediately to the regional neurological center. I had surgery 5 days later. The surgeon was able to remove only about 25% of the growth because the tumor mimicked the appearance of the brain, and in places he was unable to differentiate between tumor and healthy brain tissue. I was ultimately diagnosed with a grade III anaplastic astrocytoma and referred to a cancer center for treatment.

In the early days, it was sometimes very disheartening, especially as we learned more about this disease. In particular, while the Internet can be a tremendous source of information, it can also contain information that may be misleading. One of the scarier things to read about was the survival statistics, which can seem very grim. I made a conscious decision not to even think about them, and I encourage anyone going through a brain tumor to do the same. We are not statistics.

On November 17, I began a treatment regimen of radiation and chemotherapy together. I had radiation treatments Monday to Friday and took a low dose of Temodar 7 days a week. Other than the loss of my hair, the biggest effect was increased fatigue. Also, the steroids I was taking to relieve headaches and pressure in my brain caused bloating and affected my sleep patterns.

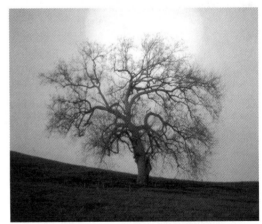

After a four-week recovery, the next phase of my treatment began, which consisted of a higher dose of Temodar for 12 months. Other than some nausea and vomiting, I tolerated the drug fairly well and my blood-level measurements stayed within acceptable limits. As much as possible, I am back to living the life I had before my diagnosis.

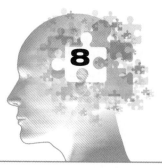

Chapter 8
Sex and fertility

Effects of treatment and medication

For patients undergoing treatment for a brain tumor, a decrease in sexual desire or in the ability to enjoy normal sexual activity is common. Deciphering the origin of these changes can be difficult, for many factors can be involved.

While surgery causes postoperative fatigue and temporary physical weakness, chemotherapy and radiation can greatly affect and reduce your desire for sexual stimulation because of adverse effects on hormone production. So, too, can medications prescribed for the symptoms of brain tumors, such as swelling, seizures, nausea, anxiety, and depression. Physical changes, such as hair loss and weight gain, can further undermine your sense of attractiveness and desirability, deepening the emotional separation from sexual contact. Individually or in various combinations, these side effects create in some cases a daunting puzzle that requires patience and communication to piece together.

Depression is common among brain tumor patients, a condition often controlled with antidepressant medication — for example, with selective serotonin reuptake inhibitors like Paxil or Zoloft. These medications can reduce sexual desire. A simple change in dosage or medication may help restore sexual desire and should be discussed with your prescribing physician.

While most treatment-associated dysfunction or lack of desire is temporary, being able to openly discuss difficulties and options for sexual intimacy with your partner and with your medical team can help in managing the extent of disruption and being able to resume normal sexual relations after treatment. Unfortunately, discomfort among health professionals in discussing sex with the same openness and honesty with which they discuss nausea, diarrhea, and even expectations for recovery can complicate your ability to understand — and prepare emotionally for — how treatment might affect sexual desire. For this reason, patients often find it beneficial to discuss issues of intimacy with other members of their medical team, such as counselors or neuropsychologists. These healthcare professionals will be familiar not only with the impact of brain trauma and the effects of medication but also with the emotional toll carried internally by the patient.

Birth control

If you take birth control pills, it is important to discuss the potential effects of your treatment with your gynecologist and with your medical team for your tumor. Chemotherapy may halt menstrual periods temporarily, but precaution against pregnancy must be maintained due to the devastating effects of chemotherapy for an unborn fetus.

Some chemotherapy medications, as well as anti-seizure drugs, can interact with the effectiveness of birth control pills. A thorough discussion with your medical care team is essential.

Sex, surgery, and brain tumor treatment

In most cases, there are few reasons why you cannot have sexual relations while undergoing radiation therapy or after surgery. However, you should always consult with your medical team regarding any precautions against strenuous activity, including sex. Both radiation therapy and surgery can result in fatigue, making any strenuous physical activity difficult. As your strength returns, normal sexual activity can resume.

Likewise, unless your medical team specifically warns you against sexual activity while undergoing chemotherapy, normal relations are limited only by the precautions associated with the drugs themselves. Because chemotherapy drugs can be transferred through sperm, in some cases they can also be harmful to sperm and also damage a fetus. Condoms should thus always be used during both intercourse and oral sex to eliminate the possibility of exposing another person either vaginally or orally to the harmful effects of chemotherapy drugs. Because sperm can live for up to three months, condoms should be used until three months have passed since the last chemotherapy treatment. Although dry orgasms can occur naturally on occasion as men age, chemotherapy can also cause this syndrome. The lack of ejaculation during orgasm is not cause for alarm and should have no adverse effect on pleasure.

Women receiving chemotherapy must take extra precaution against pregnancy, for birth defects can result from these drugs. Discuss your method of birth control with your medical team and be sure to specifically discuss whether there might be any possible reduction in the effectiveness of your birth control pills during chemotherapy. Chemotherapy can also dry out mucus membranes within the nose, mouth, and vaginal area. Non-petroleum over-the-counter vaginal lubricants can assist with the temporary dryness associated with chemotherapy, relieving the discomfort and pain often experienced during sexual relations while on chemotherapy. Because petroleum-based products can irritate the vaginal area and also weaken condoms, they should be avoided.

Fertility

Radiation to the head, surgery, and most medications (except chemotherapy drugs) used to treat brain tumors do not pose a threat to fertility. If radiation therapy is aimed at locations other than the head, you should consult your radiation oncologist about fertility concerns prior to beginning treatment. Often, a lead apron can provide adequate protection to sex organs during radiation treatments.

Chemotherapy can have a real and permanent effect on fertility in men, reducing or eliminating sperm production. While this effect is reversible in most cases, it may be a number of years before sperm counts return to normal.

In women, chemotherapy can temporarily halt menstrual periods, but normal menses should resume after treatments are concluded. Alkylating agents, however, can affect egg production (effects worsen for older women), so concerns regarding fertility should be discussed prior to beginning treatment.

The importance of fertility is a personal choice. While it is not always the priority of the medical team who are basing their treatment on life-saving measures, it should be discussed before beginning any form of chemotherapy. If necessary, you should insist on having that discussion.

Fertility experts can provide advice about the possibility of sperm banking for men or egg harvesting and fertilization techniques for women. Sperm banks typically suggest a minimum sperm count to be frozen for use at a later date, but a low count alone should not discourage you. A fertility expert can give guidance regarding your chances of success in the case of a low sperm count and other options available to you.

Although rarely the result of brain tumor treatments, impotence can occur as a result of depression. If you experience more than the occasional sexual dysfunction that is normal with aging, you should consult your medical team about medications and other available treatment avenues.

Fertility experts or physicians/therapists dealing with sexual problems near you can be located by visiting the professional societies:

- The American Medical Association (apps.ama-assn.org/doctorfinder/home.jsp)
- The American Society for Reproductive Medicine (www.asrm.org)
- The American Association of Sex Educators, Counselors, and Therapists (www.aasect.org) ●

KEY POINTS

☑ For brain tumor patients, a decrease in sexual desire is not uncommon.

☑ Discussing issues of sexual intimacy with your partner and with members of your medical team will be key to resuming normal sexual relations.

☑ If you are in your child-bearing years, talk to your doctors about using birth control and consider sperm banks or egg harvesting.

☑ Chemotherapy can produce birth defects. Use contraceptive protection.

☑ Chemotherapy can reduce fertility in both men and women.

Survivor story #8

In April 1989, asked by the girls' softball coach to demonstrate a slide (I had played softball in high school and college), I spent an afternoon practicing and banged my head on the gym floor. I was 27 years old at the time, living at home with my parents, recently engaged to the love of my life. My family physician told me to rest, but I was suffering migraines and was very tired.

The following Thursday I drove home from work with a friend. During the drive, I had another migraine, but this time the left side of my body was going numb. We went straight to the emergency room, where I was told that I should see a neurologist.

In the meantime, my mother had spoken to a neurosurgeon at a major medical center. She described my signs and symptoms, and he told her to have me carry over my CT scans to him. When he looked at them, he told me that I had a cyst that needed to be removed. I wanted to wait until after my wedding (avoiding a shaved head), but he insisted that the cyst be removed right away.

On May 2, 1989, the neurosurgeon did a craniotomy and removed a cystic astrocytoma from my right frontal lobe. The procedure was minor compared to the drug allergies I developed, and I used phenobarbital for a year to prevent seizures. I opted to not receive radiation therapy for there was no guarantee that the tumor would not reoccur. My husband to be and I wanted to start having children; our physicians felt that the tumor had been sufficiently well contained within the cyst. Wasting no time, we began trying right away to conceive a child.

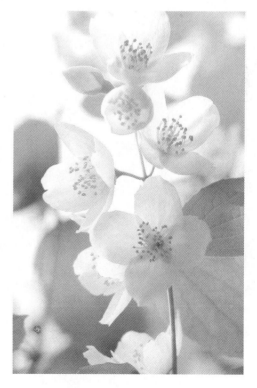

In January when I went for an MRI scan, my pregnancy test was positive. Two more children followed. My neurologist retired. When I met my new neurologist, he shockingly asked whether my husband was ready to raise our children without me. He stated that no one survives the type of brain tumor I had. My husband and I were then contemplating having a fourth child, and I had mentioned that to the new neurologist. He felt we were being foolish.

That's when I discovered the virtualtrials.com website of the Musella Foundation. I went on a rampage to learn more about brain tumors than I ever cared to know. I read many articles and emails. Some made me laugh, some made me cry. It is all such real-life stuff.

I fired the neurologist and spoke with my former neurologist, telling him that I needed a physician that knew that I was going to survive. We had a fourth child.

Since the removal of the tumor 14 years ago, I am alive and well — or as well as I can be right now. My town, home, and business were ravaged by Hurricane Sandy. The storm damage and consequent financial worry have been much worse than the storm itself, reminding me again of how many things lie outside our control. As before, I am getting through this crisis one day at a time, prayerfully. In fact, I often say to myself and others, "Hey, I survived a brain tumor … I can get through this, too."

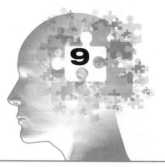

Chapter 9
"Real-world" and online support groups

Support groups found on the Internet or a local support group sponsored by your hospital/ regional cancer organization can often assist with nonmedical issues — such as nutrition, relationships, and/or financial concerns.

Most people are shy about joining a support group, but don't be. You will be amazed at how quickly you feel at ease, because the members know and understand what you are going through, something (hopefully) nobody else in your circle of friends knows about.

"Real-world" support groups

We urge all brain tumor patients to try out one or several support groups, whether online or "real world." It is a very powerful experience to speak directly with people who have undergone the same passage. Real-world and even online support groups are typically facilitated by nurses or other caregivers.

If you live near a metropolitan area, you can attend a support group in person. These support groups provide community, and they can be safe places to open up and share both positive and negative emotions.

Some cancer and dedicated brain tumor organizations provide search engines on their websites that can help you find nearby real-world support groups in your area. These organizations include:

- **American Brain Tumor Association**. Go to: www.abta.org/brain-tumor-treatment/ brain-tumor-support/support-group.

- **Cancer Care**. This organization is a national leader in providing professional services to help people manage the emotional and financial challenges of cancer. Visit: www.cancercare.org.

9

- **The National Brain Tumor Society**. Go to: www.brain-tumor-information/finding-support-coping.

The Musella Foundation provides a comprehensive list of "real-world" face-to-face support groups, with contact numbers and email addresses, and with meeting locations and schedules. To access that list to find a support group near where you live, go to: www.virtualtrials.com/support.cfm.

Online support groups

The Internet and social media sites offer an unlimited resource for brain tumor patients, including online support groups, sometimes called "mailing lists" or "listservs," chat groups, and message boards for sharing experiences and treatment options with others who understand what you're going through. Although social media sites like Facebook are a good way to keep in touch with family and friends, and some brain-tumor groups are active there, be aware that Facebook is very public. So be cautious, and be sure to activate privacy settings, if you do not want information about yourself or your medical condition to be available for years to people who do not know you.

Below is a listing of online support groups that are run by the Musella Foundation:

- **Braintumor treatments group.** Our main brain tumor online support group. Talk is limited to medical discussions about brain tumor treatments (as well as diagnoses, testing, symptoms, etc.). Discussion about all types of brain tumors is allowed: malignant, benign, primary, and metastatic. No talk of politics, jokes, religion allowed. For those, use the other groups listed below.
- **Brain tumor Novocure group.** For people interested in the Optune device.
- **Acoustic neuroma group.**
- **Brain tumor faith group.** For discussions involving faith, religion, and God among people interested in brain tumors.
- **Optic glioma group.**
- **Brainstem glioma group.** Adults and children with brainstem tumors.

There are many other online support groups for brain tumor patients that are not run or endorsed by the Musella Foundation but are listed at the virtualtrials.com website.

A word of caution: Support groups (both online and "real world") play an important and, in many cases, vital role in maintaining a positive outlook during treatment, as well as staying up-to-date on the latest brain tumor issues. However, you have to be cautious and evaluate how much you can trust anything you find. There are bad people out there looking to make money off of your misfortune, and even people who are trying to help might inadvertently supply you with misleading information. NOTHING on the Internet or at a support group meeting should be taken as medical advice. You have to research anything you find and discuss it with your medical team. Chat rooms are most susceptible to problems because there may be very few other people online with whom you can discuss the pros and cons of a treatment. On the other hand, in an online support group like the "Braintumor treatments group," you can ask for the experiences of many people with a specific treatment and get a broader view of it.

When using the Internet, exercise common sense and discuss information with your medical team to help you make the best possible decisions about your care. To evaluate information found on a website, consider the credentials of the person posting the information, how up-to-date the site is, whether any contact information is posted on the site, and whether the claims on the site are too good to be true or sound as if something is being sold to you. ●

There are many online support groups with different focuses. The Musella Foundation runs and manages a number of online support groups, and it maintains a list of many other online support groups. To see what is available, go to: www.virtualtrials.com/lists.cfm.

9

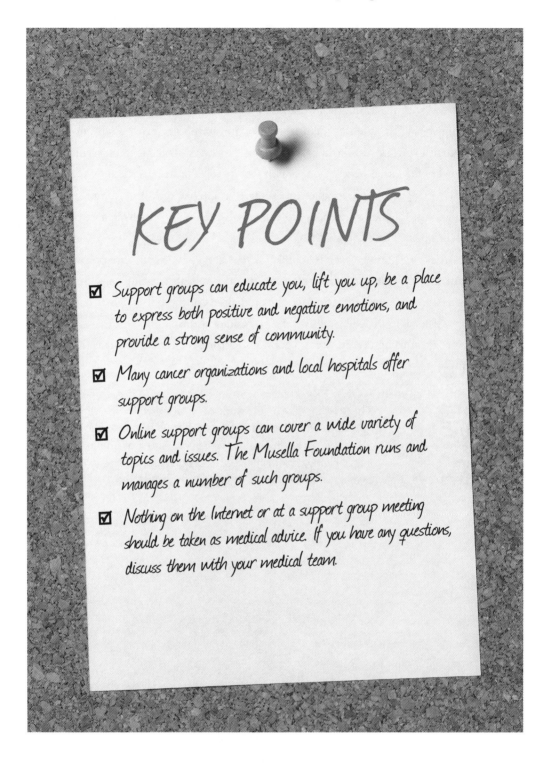

KEY POINTS

☑ Support groups can educate you, lift you up, be a place to express both positive and negative emotions, and provide a strong sense of community.

☑ Many cancer organizations and local hospitals offer support groups.

☑ Online support groups can cover a wide variety of topics and issues. The Musella Foundation runs and manages a number of such groups.

☑ Nothing on the Internet or at a support group meeting should be taken as medical advice. If you have any questions, discuss them with your medical team.

Survivor story #9

In June 2000, when I was 33 years old, my life quickly changed. I began having head-aches that felt as if my skull were going to explode. An MRI scan showed that my brain was hemorrhaging, and I went immediately into surgery. An acorn-sized glioblastoma multiforme (GBM) tumor was found in my left temporal lobe. I was told I had less than a year to live.

I quit my job to be a stay-at-home mom, wanting to spend every precious moment with my boys. I went into conformal brain radiation. I refused chemotherapy because standard treatment at that time had seriously bad side effects and would only add a few months to my life.

In July 2004, the GBM came back. I had "awake" surgery since the GBM was located in my left temporal lobe and there was a high risk of my losing the ability to speak. After surgery I went on the 5-day, 23-week Temodar schedule.

Again the GBM came back. I went into brain surgery a third time. The tumor was only the size of a "pea," but during surgery a buffer around the tumor was removed. After surgery I again went back on Temodar.

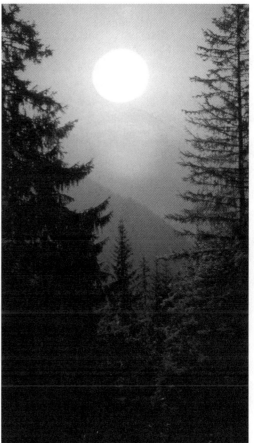

In March 2009, the GBM came back once more. This time the tumor was not even located in my brain but in the meninges (the layer of tissue that covers the brain). I went into surgery a fourth time and all "visible" tumor was removed. The brain itself looked nice and clear, no visible tumor in the brain itself. After surgery, I could not go back on Temodar since it had quit working for me, and I did not qualify for any clinical trials because of the third reoccurrence of the cancer and my treatment his-tory. We decided to keep an eye on the tumor with MRI scans every 2 months.

It's now been more than 12 years since my first battle with GBM, and these have been the best years of my

9

life! I have been blessed to see my boys grow. During these years, connecting with others battling brain tumors has inspired me so much. Al Musella and the virtualtrials.com website have been so helpful. Reading survivor stories is encouraging. Please don't feel it is over. Don't listen to the statistics. We can still love life and have fun even as brain tumor patients.

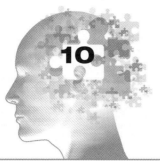

Chapter 10
Insurance management and financial assistance

Insurance under the Patient Protection and Affordable Care Act

Some people with brain tumors are afraid that their health insurance will be cancelled because they have become sick. Others are afraid that the cost of their medical treatment during a year or over a lifetime will exceed dollar pay-out limits set by their health insurance plan, thereby depleting life savings or even bankrupting them. Others are afraid that if they lose their job — and the health insurance that goes with the job — while being treated for a brain tumor, they will not be able to find new health insurance because of the preexisting condition. Or they are afraid that they will not be able to afford the health insurance even if they can continue with their existing policy or if they do find new coverage.

The Patient Protection and Affordable Care Act (ACA), the federal law passed in 2010 and being fully put into effect now, was enacted to help displace such fears. Many national cancer organizations have evaluated the ACA. According to the American Cancer Society, for example, the ACA has helped and will help people with brain tumors in the following ways:

• Upon passage, the law immediately stopped insurance companies from dropping patients from coverage just because they got sick.

• Upon passage, the law immediately banned health insurance companies from having lifetime pay-out limits. In 2014, the law banned health insurance companies from having annual pay-out limits.

• Upon passage, the law immediately banned health insurance companies from denying coverage to children with preexisting conditions. In 2014, the law banned health insurance companies from denying coverage to adults with preexisting conditions, like cancer.

• Upon passage, the law immediately banned health insurance companies from denying coverage to patients who participate in clinical trials.

• Upon passage, the law immediately banned health insurance companies from charging patients for cancer screening tests, such as mammograms and colonoscopies.

• In 2014, the law required all states to create online health insurance marketplaces (usually called "exchanges") so that people without insurance through employment can compare and buy coverage from health insurance companies. If states decided not to establish an exchange for itself, the federal government implemented an exchange for the state. The law also required that people who cannot afford health care insurance through their state exchange receive financial help to do so.

With passage of the ACA, if you had health insurance through your employment, you kept your current health insurance. However, your health insurance plan now has to abide by the provisions of the ACA law, such as following the ban on lifetime and annual pay-out limits and providing free cancer-screening tests, among others.

The American Brain Tumor Association has created and continually updates a comprehensive primer about how the Affordable Care Act will affect patients with brain tumors. To access this resource, go to: www.abta.org/care-treatment/support-resources/the-affordable-care-act.html.

The costs of cancer care

Even with insurance coverage, cancer care can be expensive and result in financial hardship. Many people have insurance plans with yearly deductibles, specified amounts of expenses they must pay out of pocket each year before the insurance plan will begin paying any costs. After the yearly deductible is met, insurance plans also often require co-insurance payments. For example, with a typical 80/20 co-insurance rate, the insurance plan will pay 80% of approved medical costs while the patients must pay the remaining 20% of medical costs out of pocket. Finally, many insurance plans require copayments. A copayment is a set fee, like $30, that an insurance plan requires the patient to pay out of pocket each time the patient visits a physician.

Consequently, taking into account deductibles, co-insurance payments, and copayments, the amount of out-of-pocket costs for direct medical care — visits to physicians, surgery, radiation therapy, chemotherapy — can add up to a considerable amount even for patients with excellent insurance plans.

But in addition to direct medical costs, there are also many nonmedical expenses associated with cancer treatment. These include transportation, hotels, meals, and childcare.

In a recent issue of the medical journal *Neuro-Oncology Practice,* investigators analyzed the out-of-pocket expenses for 43 patients diagnosed with malignant glioma between August 2008 and May 2012. Of these 43 patients, 35 (81%) were newly diagnosed with malignant glioma. The majority had private medical insurance; 10 (23%) had Medicare or Medicaid coverage, and 2 (5%) were uninsured. The investigators found that the monthly median out-of-pocket expense for these patients was $1342 (remember, the median is the middle value in a set of measurements, with half the values above that middle value and half below). Within that monthly median out-of-pocket amount, the highest components were payments for medication ($710), hospital bills ($403), and transportation ($327). These expenses decreased after 3 months, suggesting that expenses were reduced after the completion of radiation therapy. The investigators also found that median lost wages were $7500 and that median lost work time was 12.8 days.

After this study was conducted, the Affordable Care Act went fully into effect, with the availability of exchanges. In addition, in November 2013, Temodar became available as a less expensive generic drug. Nonetheless, patients and families need to be aware that cancer care can be expensive.

Understanding your insurance

Insurance laws vary from state to state. Also, your health insurance policy may be under state or federal guidelines depending on where you work and whether your employer is self-insured. A large employer who is self-insured is not considered an insurance company but rather writes its own policy that is in turn managed by an oversight organization, which may be a health maintenance organization (HMO) operating within your state. The self-insured policies are governed by federal laws, and even state laws such as in California — with strict HMO laws protecting consumers — are not available to those covered by self-insured federally regulated plans.

Complicating things even further, plans such as HMOs and preferred provider organizations (PPOs) often fall under different jurisdictions as well. Your human resources department at your employer can often tell you if your plan is self-insured, whether it is governed by state or by federal regulations, and the contact information for the proper agency.

10

Most insurance plans contain a specific list of "covered" medications and those that are excluded from coverage, called a "formulary," and by law must provide you with a copy upon request. Many of the drugs used in the treatment of brain tumors are approved by the FDA for other conditions but are not approved for treatment of conditions associated with brain tumors. When a physician prescribes a medication for a condition that falls outside the FDA approved guidelines, it's called an "off-label" use, and in many cases is not covered.

Many states provide an appeal process for challenging an off-label denial that may assist you in obtaining coverage. You may be required (if for no other reason than your immediate need of the drug) to pay for the prescription out of pocket, as the process may take several weeks for a decision. If your employer or the insurance company will allow you to upgrade your prescription coverage to one that will allow for off-label medication coverage, you would be wise to do so now, regardless of whether or not you require such coverage at this time — it's likely you will need it in the future.

Note: Request a copy of your insurance plan's formulary and keep it in your treatment binder. Have your physician check the formulary when prescribing a new medication to ensure coverage, or perhaps select a like drug (if available) from the formulary to avoid unnecessary out-of-the-pocket expense.

Information regarding the laws that govern switching plans during treatment or "continuity of care" issues when policies change with new employment can best be answered by calling your state's insurance commissioner office. Many states, such as California, have specific departments for patient advocacy that can help you work through these issues, or direct you to the proper federal agency if your plan is governed by federal regulations. Such patient advocates within your state health insurance department can also help you file the necessary paperwork for appealing denials of coverage from your insurance company for specific treatments or medications, or to file complaints.

The following are some tips for dealing with insurance companies:

- All communications (from making claims to general inquiries) should be in writing.
- When communicating by phone or in person, be sure to record and confirm your understanding of the conversation in a letter sent certified with confirmation of receipt, and keep a copy of the letter in your file.
- Scrutinize everything you receive from the insurance company and hospital — for example, bills, payments, and credits for mistakes — they DO happen! Do not be afraid to ask for explanations for items that are unclear or unspecified.
- Read your policy thoroughly so that you are aware of what benefits you are entitled to and what items are excluded, paying special attention to areas involving clinical trials or experimental treatments. Be prepared to ask your physician to write a letter

on your behalf explaining why you should be allowed coverage for these items. It is helpful to have an "understanding" with your physician as to when consideration of experimental therapies would take place, rather than waiting for that day to arrive, only to find an unsupportive care partner.

- Health insurance companies can assign a case manager to you so that you can talk to the same person each time you call. Ask your insurance company whether you can be assigned a case manager.

- Do not hesitate to ask to deal with a "superior" of the person handling your account, and keep accurate information regarding the names of all persons (and their positions) involved with your claims.

- Before making a request, make sure that the person you are dealing with has the authority to grant it.

- Do not be intimidated.

- Do not hesitate to challenge anything that doesn't sound right to you.

- If you are unsure about anything, check with the State Insurance Department (see above) and then, if necessary, with a lawyer. If you do not think you can afford a lawyer, you may be able to get low-cost or free legal help. Try calling the local bar association to ask about legal aid (available through nonprofit organizations in most major communities) or a local law school to ask if they have a student law clinic.

- Most states have nonprofit advocacy organizations dedicated to access and continuity of care issues, able to discuss your legal rights and avenues for contesting insurance decisions on your behalf. You can search the Internet using the words: insurance denials, HMO, continuity of care, or healthcare access along with "patient advocates." In California, Citizens for the Right to Know is an excellent resource.

- Set up and keep a file of all correspondence and phone communications relating to your claims. The file should include, but not be limited to, bills, payments, claims, letters you send, letters you receive, checks, contacts, and your policy.

- Be sure that all of your premiums are paid on time. You may have trouble getting insurance again if you let your policy lapse.

- Keep track of all of your unreimbursed medical expenses. You might be able to claim these expenses on your tax returns.

The American Society of Clinical Oncology sponsors a website for patients called Cancer.net This website has an excellent section on financial considerations related to cancer care, including a video presentation. Especially relevant is the page entitled "Questions to Ask about Cost." Go to: www.cancer.net/navigating-cancer-care/financial-considerations.

10

Financial assistance

There are many organizations and even individuals that provide financial assistance to patients with brain tumors and their families. Miles for Hope, for example, provides flight assistance to those participating in clinical trial treatment. Other organizations might not provide direct help with expenses but can help reduce the costs associated with medical care. Angel Flight was created by a group of volunteer pilots to provide for free air transportation for medically related needs when time is important but the trip is not an emergency. The organization called Mission4Maureen has funds to cover an array of expenses, from travel for treatment, to maintaining a place to live, to paying medical bills not covered by insurance.

The Musella Foundation runs a co-pay assistance program for people with health insurance for one or more of the following treatments: Avastin, Gliadel wafer, Temodar, and the Optune device. To find out about this program, go to: https://braintumorcopays.org/index.cfm.

The Musella Foundation runs two different programs to help you with treatment costs. For people with insurance, we have *a co-pay assistance program* for one or more of the following treatments: Avastin, Gliadel wafer, Temodar, and the Optune device.

For people without insurance, we have a *Musella Foundation Drug Discount Card* that can save everyone — not just patients with brain tumors — up to 80% or more off the cost of prescription medicines, over-the-counter medicines (that is, medicines not needing a prescription), and even prescription medicines for pets. There is no cost for the card, there is no risk in using it, and it is immediately available online, with no registration required. You take the card to your pharmacy and ask how much the prescription would cost using this card compared with how much it would cost without it. If using the card is less expensive for the prescription, then use it.

The Musella Foundation provides a Musella Foundation Drug Discount Card for all patients, but especially those patients without insurance. To get the card immediately, go to: www.virtualtrials.com/drug_assistance.cfm.

The Musella Foundation Drug Discount Card can also be used by patients who have insurance — but you cannot combine the discount this card provides with the discount your insurance provides. Sometimes the card discount will be greater than your insurance discount.

Here is a list of other organizations that can help you.

• **American Brain Tumor Association** (www.abta.org/care-treatment/support-resources/financial-medical-assistance.html)

• **Angel Flight Travel Assistance** (www.angelflight.com)

• **Cancer Care** (www.cancercare.org)

• **Drug Assistance Programs from Pharmaceutical Companies** (www.cancersupportivecare.com/drug_assistance.html)

• **Medicare Rights Center** (www.medicarerights.org)

• **Medicare Prescription Drug Program** (www.medicare.gov)

• **Miles for Hope Travel Assistance** (www.milesforhope.org)

• **Mission for Maureen Travel Assistance** (www.mission4maureen.org)

• **NeedyMeds** (www.needymeds.org)

• **Patient Advocate Foundation** (www.copays.org)

• **Supplemental Security Income (SSI) & Social Security Disability Insurance** (www.socialsecurity.gov/)

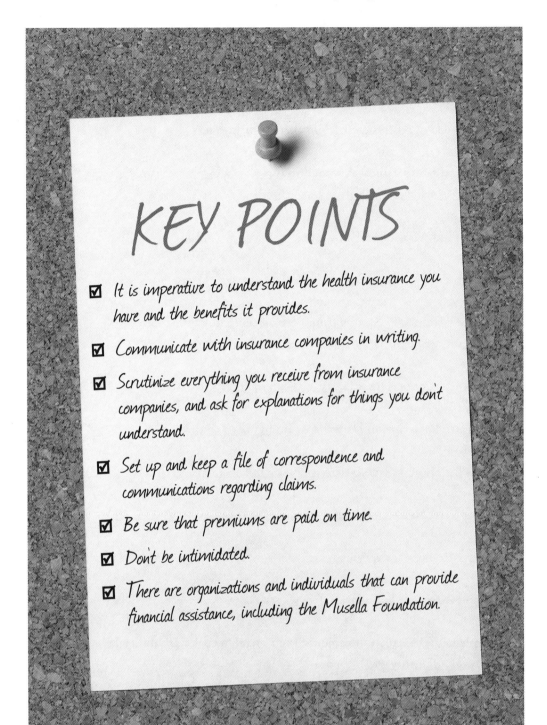

KEY POINTS

☑ It is imperative to understand the health insurance you have and the benefits it provides.

☑ Communicate with insurance companies in writing.

☑ Scrutinize everything you receive from insurance companies, and ask for explanations for things you don't understand.

☑ Set up and keep a file of correspondence and communications regarding claims.

☑ Be sure that premiums are paid on time.

☑ Don't be intimidated.

☑ There are organizations and individuals that can provide financial assistance, including the Musella Foundation.

Survivor story #10

On June 1, 2005, just five weeks after the birth of my first child, I was diagnosed with glioblastoma multiforme (GBM). This malignant and deadly type of brain tumor was the size of a woman's fist. GBM patients are told that "it's not a matter of if, it's a matter of when" the tumor will come back.

I quickly underwent brain surgery to remove the GBM. The problem with brain surgery is that the doctors don't know what they will find until they cut into your head and take a look. After discovering that removing the tumor could cause a loss of mobility on my left side, the surgeons removed only half of it. I was told I would be lucky to live a year. I kept telling the doctors that that couldn't be right, because I had just had my first child.

My husband and I were not going to give up easily. We hit the road to visit some prestigious cancer centers after receiving the worst possible pathology report. Both brain tumor clinics recommended that I "re-do" my brain surgery to complete the removal of the tumor. I chose one of these centers to coordinate all of my treatment. I also went on long-term disability to cover my medical bills and keep my business afloat.

In July 2005, surgeons operated again to remove the remaining tumor, a procedure that was successful.

At that time, I entered a clinical trial that involved the implantation of a drug locally at the affected areas in my brain, treatment that required a four-day stay in a neuro-intensive care unit. Most brain surgeries remove the tumor but not all the damaged cells. The new procedure was a way to kill off the remaining damaged cells and prevent the tumor from coming back. I was lucky that my health insurance paid for the hospital stay and all expenses. Frequently, we had no idea whether our health insurance would pay for an experimental treatment if needed.

The surgeries and experimental drug procedure were a success. Nonetheless, I lost a lot of my cognitive function, and it took weeks for me to recover.

As if the brain surgeries weren't enough, my family and I moved to the location of the cancer center to receive a complete series of radiation treatment. After radiation, I then began a year of chemotherapy. I returned to work during this important recovery period. Because of my disability insurance, I didn't have to come back to work, but I love what I do. But without the disability income, I would not have been able to keep my business afloat. It was a life saver.

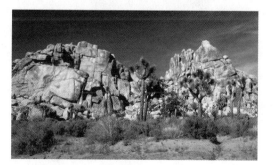

10

Afterword

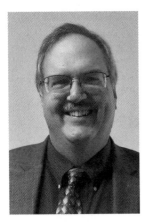

Al Musella, DPM

In 1992, my sister-in-law Lana, a mother with four children, was diagnosed with glioblastoma multiforme (GBM). Lana had surgery and radiation, but then the first MRI scan after radiation showed that the tumor had grown even larger. This was before Temodar, the Gliadel wafer, and Avastin were available. So the outlook for Lana was bleak. Also, because at that time there was no centralized database of clinical trials for brain tumor patients, we could not readily find clinical trials for her to enter.

But I was a computer geek. I started the first online support group dedicated to brain tumors on Compuserv and AOL. I also published a brain-tumor clinical trials database online, one of the first database-driven websites for any cancer type. Lana found that she was eligible for many clinical trials and tried two of them. She did much better than expected. She lived eight years, a survival course that was almost unheard of back then, and for most of that time she remained in good health.

In 1998, the Musella Foundation was organized as a not-for-profit charity dedicated to speeding up the search for cures of brain tumors and to helping families deal with the diagnosis of brain tumor. Ironically, my father was diagnosed with GBM the very next year. We were more prepared than previously to deal with this diagnosis, but it was still a horrendous experience to go through. Because his tumor progressed so rapidly, my father died only a few months after it was discovered.

Since then, a lot has been accomplished by the Musella Foundation:

- Our virtualtrials.com website continues to expand in terms of services provided and the community served (in 2015 we had 890,000 visitors from 231 different countries).

- In the first three years of operation of our direct co-payment assistance program, we have awarded almost $3 million to brain tumor patients.

- We created and run the Brain Tumor Virtual Trial, our study of brain tumor patients, as well as the long-term glioblastoma multiforme outcome project.

- We helped convince Medicare to pay for Temodar and for Gliadel wafers, and we are working on getting Medicare to pay for Optune. We have helped accelerate FDA approval of Temodar, Avastin, and Optune for brain tumors.

- Along with the Brad Kaminsky Foundation and a group called Unlocking Brain Tumors, we co-founded the Heroes of Hope Grey Ribbon Crusade, which has involved over 60 brain tumor foundations working together to help fund research projects.

Most important, we think, are the online support groups that we run. Every family dealing with a brain tumor should have at least one member join the "Braintumor treatments group" through our website. Joining that group allows you to communicate with more than 2600 families going through the same passage. Those who have travelled further down that road can help — and want to help — those of you starting out right now.

In the 24 years that I have been immersed in the world of brain tumors, I have seen an amazing change in attitude among brain tumor researchers. There has been an unprecedented burst of progress in identifying new approaches. I am convinced that we are in the home stretch, that a cure is within sight. It is now only a matter of time and money. But although the government now funds brain tumor research at an unprecedented level, many promising projects remain unfunded. Through the Musella Foundation, we have a chance to speed up the search for a cure, by funding selected research that complements, without duplicating, research funded by the government.

To that end, we need your help. Donations to the Musella Foundation can be general or can be dedicated to specific ends, like our support for brain tumor research or our copayment assistance program. For more details on how you can help us speed up the search for the cure, please visit the virtualtrials.com website. ●

Al Musella, DPM
Founder and President
The Musella Foundation for Brain Tumor Research and Information

Recent grants made by the Musella Foundation

Below is a listing of recent research grants made by the Musella Foundation. Since 2003, the Musella Foundation has awarded investigators with close to $3 million in more than 90 different grants.

Interested investigators should call the Musella Foundation directly to discuss the project(s) for which they seek funding before submitting the formal grant application.

To see a list of all grants awarded by the Musella Foundation, please go to the grants page at the virtualtrials.com website (www.virtualtrials.com/grants.cfm).

Grants awarded to date in 2016

- $50,000 to investigators at Cold Spring Harbor Laboratory, Cold Spring Harbor, New York, for the project "Antisense therapy for pediatric diffuse intrinsic pontine glioma (DIPG)," to which the DIPG Consortium, Edgewater, New Jersey has added another $50,000.

- $49,992 to investigators at Duke University Medical Center, Durham, North Carolina for the project "Phase I study of oncolytic polio/rhinovirus recombinant against recurrent malignant glioma in children."

- $50,000 to investigators at the Yale School of Engineering and Applied Sciences, New Haven, Connecticut, for the project "Convection-enhanced delivery of drug-loaded nanoparticles for the treatment of glioblastoma multiforme."

- $50,000 to investigators at Ohio State University, Columbus, Ohio, for the project "Combined stereotactic radiation and immunotherapy in CNS gliomas."

- $5,000 to investigators at the Medical College of Wisconsin, Milwaukee, Wisconsin, for the project "Development of acid ceramidase inhibitors and tumor vaccine against glioblastoma and medulloblastoma."

- $5,000 to the Central Brain Tumor Registry of the United States, Hinsdale, Illinois, to help further their vital mission of gathering and disseminating brain-tumor epidemiologic data.

- $8,000 to investigators at Duke University Medical Center, Durham, North Carolina, for the project "Targeting GBMs with activated EGFR with third-generation brain-penetrating AZD9291."

Grants awarded in 2015

- $32,500 to investigators at the CHOP Research Institute in Philadelphia, Pennsylvania, for the project "Cytokine, RNA, and proteonomic analyses of the immune response to a molecular targeted therapy for medulloblastoma." This grant was made in partnership with The Gray Matters Brain Cancer Foundation, which added another $32,500 for this research project.

- $50,000 to investigators at the Medical College of Wisconsin, Milwaukee, Wisconsin, for the project "Development of acid ceramidase inhibitors and tumor vaccine against glioblastoma."

- $50,000 to investigators at the Rose Ella Burkhardt Brain Tumor & Neuro-Oncology Center at the Cleveland Clinic, Cleveland, Ohio, for the project "Targeting myeloid derived suppressor cells in recurrent glioblastoma: Phase 0/1 trial of low-dose capecitabine + bevacizumab in patients with recurrent glioblastoma."

- $5,000 to investigators at Children's Hospital of Philadelphia, Philadelphia, Pennsylvania, for the project "Genomic analysis of DIPG."

- $5,000 to the Central Brain Tumor Registry of the United States, Hinsdale, Illinois, to help further their vital mission of gathering and disseminating brain-tumor epidemiologic data.

- $5,000 to investigators at JFK Neuroscience Center, Edison, New Jersey, for the project "Quality-of-care measures study for high-grade glioma."

- $25,000 to investigators at Stanford University, Palo Alto, California, for the project "Using ferumoxytol-enhanced MRI to assess tumor-associated macrophages in human glioblastoma multiforme."

- $25,000 to investigators at the University of Illinois College of Medicine, Chicago, Illinois, for the project "Preclinical studies on a p53-mediated cell-cycle inhibitor for treatment of glioblastoma."

- $50,000 to investigators at the Dana Farber Cancer Institute, Boston, Massachusetts, for the project "In vivo discovery of shRNAs that enhance the anti-tumor function of human CAR-modified T cells in glioblastoma."

- $80,000 to investigators at Tocagen, Inc., San Diego, California, for the project "Evaluation of the biocompatibility of Toca 511 with emerging modalities [5-aminolevulinic acid (5-ALA) and tumor-treating fields (TTF)] for use in treatment of high-grade glioma."

- $25,000 to the DIPG Consortium, Edgewater, New Jersey, for funding research into pediatric diffuse intrinsic pontine glioma.

- $5,000 to investigators at the Children's Research Institute, Washington, DC, for the project "Pediatric brain tumor biorepository (for DIPG specimens)."

Grants awarded in 2014

- $20,000 to investigators at Wake Forest Medical Center, Winston-Salem, North Carolina, for the project "MMP-cleavable F10 hydrogels for preventing GBM recurrence."

- $5,000 to the Central Brain Tumor Registry of the United States, Hinsdale, Illinois, to help further their vital mission of gathering and disseminating brain-tumor epidemiologic data.

- $10,000 to the Scott & White Healthcare Foundation, Temple, Texas, to sponsor their 2014 conference "At a turning point: Novel therapeutic developments in glioblastoma multiforme (GBM) research."

- $50,000 to investigators at the Cleveland Clinic, Cleveland, Ohio, for the project "Phase 1 trial of ganetespib with radiation and temozolomide in patients with newly diagnosed high-grade glioma."

- $25,000 to investigators at the Cleveland Clinic Neuro-Oncology Center, Cleveland, Ohio, for the project "Microparticles in phase 1 trial of ganetespib with temozolomide in patients with high-grade glioma."

- $50,000 to investigators at Hackensack University Medical Center, Hackensack, New Jersey, for the project "Effect of decreased hypoxia and kinase activity on radiotherapy of GL261-luc tumors."

- $5,000 to investigators at Duke University Medical Center, Durham, North Carolina, for the project "Isolation, characterization, and effect of EGFR inhibitors on stem cells from patient-derived glioblastoma xenografts."

- $25,000 to investigators at Oncoceutics, Inc., Philadelphia, Pennsylvania, for the project "Target identification of ONC201, a first-in-class drug to treat glioblastoma."

- $50,000 to investigators at the University of California, Los Angeles, for the project "Role of the PD-1/PD-L1 co-stimulatory axis for immunotherapy of glioma."

- $10,000 to investigators at the University of California, Irvine, for the project: "Establishing an in vivo human glioma resection model for testing and validating therapeutic effect of EFEMP1-derived tumor suppressive protein."

- $50,000 to investigators at the Swedish Medical Center, Seattle, Washington, for the project "Establishment of a reference laboratory for cytomegalovirus and other viral infections in glioblastoma."
- $50,000 to investigators at the University of Utah, Salt Lake City, Utah, for the project "Phase 1 trial in newly diagnosed high-grade glioma with temozolomide, radiation, and minocycline followed by adjuvant minocycline/temozolomide (D-TERMINED)."

- $5,000 to investigators at the Children's Research Institute in Washington, DC, for the project "Pediatric brain tumor biorepository (for DIPG specimens)."

Appendix. The virtualtrials.com website of the Musella Foundation

On the next two pages is a schematic site map of virtualtrials.com, the website of the Musella Foundation for Brain Tumor Research and Information.

The website is conceived to be an essential portal to the world of brain tumor treatments and organizations.

Updated weekly, the website contains a huge amount of information (which ranges in complexity from basic patient-related material to medical professional matters) and hundreds of links.

We hope you make full use of this website, including the online support groups, the co-payment assistance, the explanation of treatments, the listings of clinical trials and brain tumor centers, and more.

As noted in the first chapter of the book, we would like to hear from you. You can reach us by means of the website, or you can call us toll free at 888-295-4740 (or use our direct number 516-295-4740). The best time to call is between 10:00 AM and 6:00 PM ET Monday through Friday, and between 10:00 AM and 1:00 PM ET Saturday and Sunday. We are located in New York State.

Acknowledgments

Brain Tumor Guide for the Newly Diagnosed was written by Al Musella, DPM.

The Musella Foundation for Brain Tumor Research & Information, Inc., sponsors this book.

The Musella Foundation is a 501(c)(3) nonprofit public charity dedicated to speeding up the search for the cure of brain tumors and to helping families deal with brain tumors.

For brain tumor information, to join online support groups, or to make a donation, go to www.virtualtrials.com.

Call or email with questions or suggestions for this guide.

All proceeds from the sale of ***Brain Tumor Guide for the Newly Diagnosed*** are used to fund brain tumor research.

Updated October 4, 2016

The Musella Foundation for
Brain Tumor Research & Information, Inc.
1100 Peninsula Boulevard, Hewlett, NY 11557
888-295-4740
www.virtualtrials.com

The information provided in ***Brain Tumor Guide for the Newly Diagnosed*** and at the virtualtrials.com website reflects the diverse opinions of many different people, most of whom are not physicians or nurses trained to practice oncology, neuro-oncology, or neurosurgery.

The information in this book and at the website should therefore be considered simply as ideas for further exploration with your personal doctors. It is not offered as medical advice from any person at the Musella Foundation or associated with the book or website, and it should not be considered medical advice.

If you find any errors, disagree with what we say, or have suggestions to improve it, please contact us by email at musella@virtualtrials.com or phone toll free at 888-295-4740.

Site map of virtualtrials.com

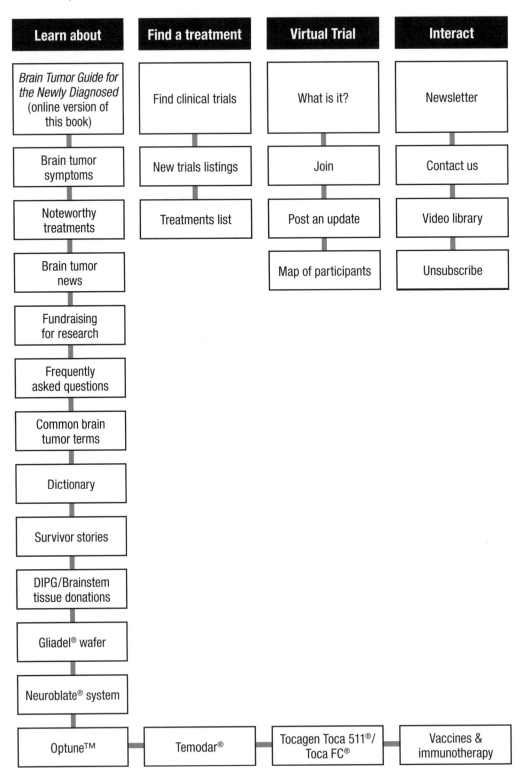

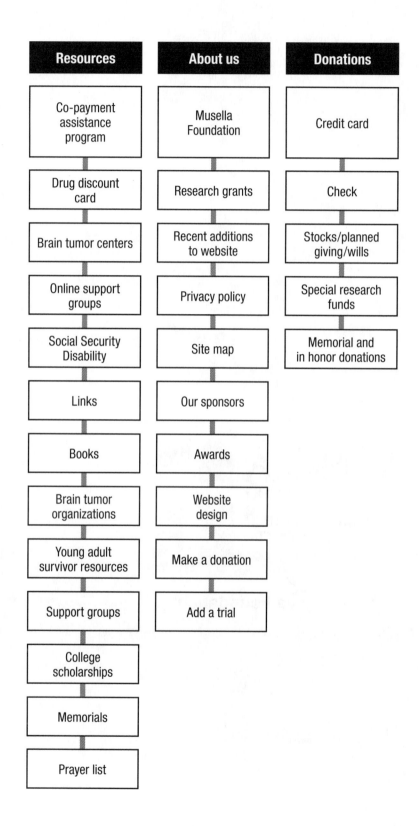

Resources	About us	Donations
Co-payment assistance program	Musella Foundation	Credit card
Drug discount card	Research grants	Check
Brain tumor centers	Recent additions to website	Stocks/planned giving/wills
Online support groups	Privacy policy	Special research funds
Social Security Disability	Site map	Memorial and in honor donations
Links	Our sponsors	
Books	Awards	
Brain tumor organizations	Website design	
Young adult survivor resources	Make a donation	
Support groups	Add a trial	
College scholarships		
Memorials		
Prayer list		

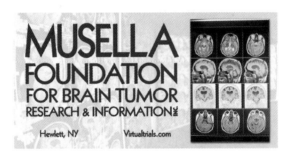

The Musella Foundation

1100 Peninsula Boulevard, Hewlett, NY 11557

888-295-4740

www.virtualtrials.com